CHOLESTEROL

CONTROL

WITHOUT

DIET!

THE NIACIN SOLUTION

CHOLESTEROL CONTROL WITHOUT DIET!

THE NIACIN SOLUTION

William B. Parsons Jr., M.D.

Lilac Press
Scottsdale, Arizona

Although the author and publisher have exhaustively researched many sources to assure the accuracy and completeness of the information contained in this book, we assume no responsibility for errors, inaccuracies, omissions or other inconsistency herein. Any slights against people or organizations are unintentional. Specifically, as the author repeatedly points out in the text, the use of niacin for cholesterol control requires knowledgeable medical supervision, even though anyone can purchase it over-the-counter, without a prescription. In the doses used to treat abnormal cholesterol levels, niacin is not a vitamin or nutritional supplement; it is a drug, with beneficial effects but with the potential for serious toxic effects if used without ongoing medical supervision.

First printing 1998

ISBN 0-9662568-6-7

LCCN 98-65160

Design, typesetting and printing services provided by About Books, Inc., 425 Cedar Street, POB 1500, Buena Vista, CO 81211, (800) 548-1876.

ATTENTION CORPORATIONS, UNIVERSITIES, COLLEGES, AND PROFESSIONAL ORGANIZATIONS: Quantity discounts are available on bulk purchases of this book for educational purposes. Special books or book excerpts can also be created to fit specific needs. For information, please contact Lilac Press, P.O. Box 1356, Scottsdale, AZ 85252-1356, phone (602) 368-8656.

ACKNOWLEDGEMENTS

The author gratefully acknowledges the following invaluable assistance and associations:

- Marihelen (Micki) O'Connor, Pat Carli, and Nita Mailander for library assistance

- Tom Bethune, R.Ph., and Greg Chavez, R.Ph. for drug price information

- Abram Hoffer, M.D. for bringing the niacin idea across the border

- The late Rudolf Altschul, M.U.Dr. for suggesting it to him

- Ken Berge, M.D., the late Dick Achor, M.D., and the late John Flinn, M.D., dear friends and co-workers in the early years

- My daughter, Dana, for permanent loan of her word processor to write "the long book" and for her illustration

- My son, Tyler, for computer guidance and trouble-shooting

- My wonderful wife, Lynn, for her near-perfect patience in tolerating the many evening and weekend hours required for me to write this book while conducting a full-time medical practice, with my apology for those many lonely times

DEDICATION

To Lynn

CONTENTS

INTRODUCTION

Everyone likes good news.
This good news should make everyone happy:

You Don't Have To Diet To Control Cholesterol!

Right! When you hear "cholesterol," you may automatically think "diet." That's because you have been brainwashed over the years by diet advocates and the food industry. The media has played a major role in brainwashing the public, but they haven't known any better—until now. This book should serve as a wake-up call for the media and the public. It can simplify life for almost everyone.

You do *not* have to diet to control cholesterol—if your doctor is good at niacin. Niacin, a drug whose use for cholesterol control I pioneered in the United States (1955) and introduced to the medical world (1956), does everything right to achieve today's goals of cholesterol control. It does so while you eat as you please!

At best, diet is a weak and often ineffective method of altering blood cholesterol levels. Drugs accomplish this purpose better, and niacin is unquestionably the best drug currently available. No other drug has all of its benefits.

If niacin treatment for cholesterol goes back more than forty years, why haven't we heard more about it? The most important reason is that niacin has never been patentable, so no company can make large profits from its exclusive sale. Therefore, niacin has had no blockbuster ad campaigns to teach physicians and the public its distinctive advantages. Besides that, die-hard advocates of diet have kept singing their tired refrain, and the unsuspecting public has accepted its message. Pharmaceutical companies

1

with patents on expensive (and less effective) products have sponsored gigantic studies, then inundated the medical profession (and lately the public as well) with multi-million dollar advertising, seeking larger shares of the multi-billion dollar market. And who has paid for all this? If you say "the drug companies," you are wrong. Those who pay are the purchasers of their expensive products, whose benefits dim by comparison with niacin.

Why is niacin better than the other drugs? To begin with, it reduces blood levels of "bad" cholesterol. Because bad cholesterol is the largest fraction, this reduces total cholesterol as well. Niacin also increases "good" cholesterol. It reduces triglycerides, if they are part of the problem. These changes all tend to reduce heart attack risk. No other drug does all of these things.

Niacin also produces favorable changes in several lesser-known cholesterol-containing fractions, which we will discuss in an early chapter. No other drug currently available produces these benefits in newly discovered cholesterol fractions. Neither does any other maneuver, such as diet or exercise.

What is the end result of these niacin-induced changes in blood cholesterol values? In a landmark study, the Coronary Drug Project (CDP), performed from 1966 to 1974, niacin reduced heart attacks, strokes and related events, cardiovascular (heart and blood vessel) surgery, cardiovascular hospitalization, all hospitalization, and deaths. None of the three other drugs studied in the CDP produced any of these benefits, and none of them is still in current use. No currently used drug has all of these favorable effects, although studies in the last few years show that a couple of drugs have some of them.

Because of all these distinctive advantages, not shared or even approached by any other cholesterol-control drugs on the market today, niacin stands alone as the drug of choice. When penicillin was first discovered, it was called a "wonder drug." In today's more sophisticated society, the term "designer drug" is more appropriate for niacin. If one lists all the desirable characteristics for a cholesterol-control drug, niacin accomplishes every goal on the "wish list." No other drug comes close.

Could there possibly be even more good news? Yes, there is. The usual cost of niacin, whether plain or time-release, is about eight to ten dollars a month. The cost of other drugs for cholesterol control can be as little as $48 a month or as great as $222 a month. In general, the other drugs cost six to ten times as much as niacin. Project this for a year in one patient: $96 to $120 for niacin, six to ten times that (about $600 to $1200) for other agents.

Niacin is available over-the-counter, without a prescription. Then, some might conclude, the proper thing to do in order to control cholesterol, to prevent heart attacks and other related events, is to buy some niacin and start taking it—right? *Absolutely not!* Here is the most important message of this book: *Niacin is not a do-it-yourself drug. It requires knowledgeable medical supervision.* You need a doctor in charge who is adept in its use—*good at niacin.*

This book teaches the reader how to be sure his doctor is good at niacin. The best way is to *give the doctor a copy of this book.* It contains not only the essentials both physician and patient need to know but also a section of medical reports and commentary, bringing the doctor more detailed information which will give him the confidence to use niacin successfully.

Both patient and physician should know as much as possible about any method of treatment. Usually the doctor knows and teaches the patient the essential information. In this instance, both can learn about niacin from this book. A patient can understand niacin's use and work with his doctor, applying their mutual knowledge.

The book is written in the same plain words that I use in my office when talking to patients. Even the section of medical details for doctors is written in this manner because I expect most readers to understand it also. If I use a medical term that is not familiar to the general public, I explain it immediately. In addition, there is a glossary of medical terms and abbreviations. To doctors, I offer no apology for using nonmedical, understandable language. They might even enjoy reading about these matters without the stilted style of medical journals. I hope physicians will use this book as a starting point to bring their patients a better understanding of cholesterol problems.

One more note regarding writing style. I am not going to say "he/she" each time I use a pronoun in a situation that could refer to either sex. Likewise, I am not going to make this manuscript gender-neutral by changing such pronouns to "persons," "people," or "individuals" in every instance. To resolve the thorny gender issue (although I can't understand why anyone finds it a problem) I will arbitrarily try to refer to a patient as "she" or "her" and a physician as "he" or "him." This is realistic for a couple of reasons. Women are better about going to doctors and taking care of their health than men, who often wait until a heart attack gets their attention. Also women are now having more heart attacks than men, 51% by latest estimates. There are still more male physicians than women physicians, although medical school classes are now about equally divided and the numbers of women in medicine are steadily increasing. I hope my gender decision will not offend anyone or distract any reader from the book's important message.

This book is intended to make the patient an intelligent consumer regarding cholesterol control. The goal is to eliminate many heart attacks and strokes while postponing others till much later in life. I would like every person to live as one who has never had a heart attack rather than living as a heart attack survivor. There is a world of difference! For any of you who have already survived heart attacks, strokes, or blood vessel surgery, the book teaches special guidelines for you, aimed at making some cholesterol deposits regress (become smaller) while slowing the formation of new deposits.

Since I brought the use of niacin for cholesterol control to the attention of the medical world more than forty years ago, it has been used increasingly in recent years. I have had the satisfaction of knowing that niacin has already prevented or delayed heart attacks and other artery-narrowing disorders in millions of people around the world. You can bring the message about niacin's use to your doctor and to your family and friends as well. Doctors can bring the good news to their patients and have probably 90% or more of those with cholesterol problems taking niacin successfully. We can all be part of a gradual but revolutionary change in cholesterol management and heart attack prevention.

Now my challenge to the media. Put aside all the brainwashing you have received over the years from diet advocates and, in recent years, from pharmaceutical manufacturers, striving to sell their expensive drugs, none of which matches niacin's efficacy or affordability. It is not your fault that you have parroted their messages and slogans in your writings, but this has, in turn, brainwashed the public. You missed the Veritas Society's symposium, which led to the book *Coronary Heart Disease: The Dietary Sense and Nonsense*, cited in these pages, but the book is still available.

I invite members of the media to read the simple truths and logic of *Cholesterol Control Without Diet!* and report them, undismayed by the howls and screams of dietary advocates and niacin detractors. You can do a great service to untold numbers of persons who, without your work, might not learn these lessons. For some, this could mean the difference between life and death, or between living as a person without a previous heart attack rather than as a heart attack survivor. You or some one close to you could be one of those beneficiaries.

To everyone: know what your bad and good cholesterol fractions are and realize that if they are both in the proper ranges, total cholesterol is really irrelevant. If either or both (bad and good cholesterol fractions) should not be in desirable ranges, work out a treatment program with your doctor, as outlined in this book. If your bad and good cholesterol fractions are now in desirable ranges without treatment, resolve to recheck them in three years. Then go on living a normal life and *enjoy every day!* As I have said in another place and time[1]: "Perhaps we can get back to basics: eat food because it tastes good, exercise because it feels good, control weight because it looks good, and be happy, because life should be enjoyed, one day at a time."

Chapters to come will answer questions which naturally occur to anyone hearing about cholesterol control by niacin for the first time—or to physicians who may have been misled by rumors that niacin is difficult to manage.

- How did niacin's use for cholesterol control get started?
- Why is it important to control cholesterol?
- How can you assess your risk factors for heart attack and apply current guidelines for treatment?
- Why not use diet to control cholesterol?
- What are the important differences between plain and time-release niacin?
- How should the doctor start treatment with either type of niacin?
- What are the side effects, and how does a doctor good at niacin manage them?
- What about the other drugs for cholesterol control?
- What can you say to your doctor to be sure that he is good at niacin?

---

[1] Final statement in my chapter, *Clinical Alternatives* from the book, *Coronary Heart Disease: The Dietary Sense and Nonsense*, edited by George V. Mann, Sc.D, M.D. for the Veritas Society. Janus Publishing Company, London, England, published the book, based on a symposium in Washington, D.C., in 1993. One can order the book from the publisher by FAX: 01144-171-636-5756, with credit card information.

Part I

THE
NIACIN
SOLUTION

CHAPTER ONE

Use of Niacin for Cholesterol Control: A Brief History

I conducted the first systematic study of niacin's use for reducing blood cholesterol levels in 1955, while in my fourth and final year of fellowship (residency) at the Mayo Clinic, Rochester, Minnesota. The suggestion that large doses of niacin might lower cholesterol levels reached me that summer through an incredible series of coincidences which lead me now to believe that it was simply meant to be.

Dr. Abram Hoffer, a psychiatrist from Regina, Saskatchewan, had given a series of lectures on schizophrenia in Rochester during a week in August 1955. At dinner on his last night in town he mentioned to Dr. Howard Rome, head of the Section on Psychiatry, that for years he had been using large doses of niacin to treat schizophrenia, believing that it helped many of his patients. Dr. Rudolf Altschul, who was Professor of Anatomy at University of Saskatchewan School of Medicine, had done some cholesterol research in rabbits. He suggested that Hoffer measure cholesterol levels, which Altschul predicted would be reduced by this treatment. When this prediction proved to be correct, Hoffer and Altschul teamed with Dr. James Stephen, laboratory director at the hospital in Regina where Hoffer practiced, to check cholesterol levels in volunteers before and after niacin, using doses of three to four grams per day. They reported their brief observations, some only 24 hours in duration, in a short letter to the editor of an obscure journal, *Archives of Biochemistry and Biophysics.*

This report probably would never have come to the attention of the medical world if Hoffer had not visited Rochester when he did and mentioned their findings to Dr. Rome. Before becoming a psychiatrist, Rome had been trained in internal medicine. He was especially interested in treatment of medical conditions with drugs since the advent of Thorazine, a relatively new breakthrough drug which was getting patients out of mental hospitals. Thus he had been a receptive listener to Hoffer's tale of a drug capable of reducing elevated cholesterol levels, known to be associated with increased risk of heart attack and stroke.

Dr. Edgar V. Allen was staff consultant on the Peripheral Vascular Service at St. Mary's Hospital that month. For years he and Howard Rome had gone duck-hunting together every fall. The fact that such good friends were on their respective hospital services at the same time and that this coincided with Hoffer's visit form part of the chain of coincidences, which ends with my presence in the room to which Dr. Rome brought the news. I was first assistant on the Vascular Service that quarter and the only one sufficiently intrigued by the niacin idea to explore it further.

Before seeing our hospital patients that morning, I was sitting in a small conference room with Dr. Allen and the three second assistants on the service when Dr. Rome knocked, entered, and asked us if we would be interested in a drug which would reduce serum cholesterol levels. Dr. Allen assured him we would be if such a drug existed. Rome then told us about his dinner conversation with Hoffer.

Niacin (then usually called *nicotinic acid* in this country) had been known as the member of the vitamin B complex which prevents the deficiency disease *pellagra* in humans and a corresponding disorder, *black tongue*, in dogs. My first thought was that a single tablet of even 50 or 100 milligrams (mg) of niacin almost immediately causes an intense hot feeling with redness of the skin, especially in the face, neck, and upper part of the body. This flush is harmless and subsides in perhaps 20 to 30 minutes. Over the years the flush had led physicians to hope that niacin might help the dizziness of Meniere's disease or increase blood flow to the brain in stroke patients. (It does neither.)

Niacinamide, a closely related compound that has the same vitamin activity as niacin, is the form usually included in vitamin preparations since it does not cause the flush. In their brief, unstructured observations, the Canadians had tried using equal doses of the amide, but it had failed to reduce cholesterol levels.

Hoffer had assured Dr. Rome that when he and his associates gave large doses of niacin (1000 mg three to four times a day), the flush lessened each day until it disappeared entirely, in an average of three to four days. Armed by this assurance and with Dr. Allen's approval, I decided to try the new treatment in several patients on the Vascular Service who had high cholesterol levels. We customarily measured cholesterol and other blood lipids as part of the admission laboratory work, even though there was no effective treatment if the results were abnormal. In those days we did not have the surgical techniques which now can be used to improve leg circulation. It was not unusual to keep patients with seriously impaired circulation in the hospital for three or four weeks, attempting to heal ulcers on the feet and avoid amputation, which frequently had to be performed above the knee. Hospital charges were very inexpensive at that time, by today's standards, permitting these long stays.

That same afternoon I sat in the rooms of four or five such patients and recounted what Dr. Rome had told us about cholesterol reduction by niacin, including the early disappearance of the flush. Each of them agreed to take the drug while in the hospital to see whether we could duplicate the Canadians' results. Then I had to inform them that the largest niacin tablet available at that time was 100 mg, which meant that they would have to take ten tablets with each meal! I asked the patients not to be troubled by the number of tablets and predicted that eventually 500 mg tablets would be marketed if the new method of treatment were successful. This prediction has proved to be correct.

After we rechecked cholesterol and other lipid determinations the next morning, these patients took 1000 mg of niacin three times a day, with their meals. The flush subsided in a few days, as predicted. When cholesterol determinations were repeated one week later, *I could not believe the marked reductions*. These reductions were maintained or even improved in the second week. At this point I shared the results with the others on the Vascular Service, but it is probably correct to say that even these striking results stirred little genuine interest among the second assistants and the consultant. (By then Dr. Edgar Hines had succeeded Dr. Allen for the final month of the quarter.) To me the results were exciting, unquestionably impressive enough to warrant a carefully structured study for a longer time.

Such a study could best be done in Rochester residents, so I approached my friend and contemporary, Dick Achor, a staff member in the section that provides care for local residents. He and another young consultant, Ken Berge, had a list of patients with hypercholesteremia whom they were following, even though there was no effective treatment. They had tried thyroid and a plant product, sitosterol, both without benefit. By phoning persons on their list, I recruited eighteen patients to take part in an outpatient study for twelve weeks, the first systematic study of the new method of treatment.

Dr. Bernard McKenzie, a Mayo laboratory chemist, joined us in this project. He had a method for separating and measuring the beta and alpha$_1$ lipoprotein, already known to be the "bad" and "good" cholesterol fractions. These fractions are now known as LDL (low density lipoprotein) cholesterol and HDL (high density lipoprotein) cholesterol, respectively. Both are important in estimating an individual's risk of coronary or other atherosclerotic disease (arterial narrowing by cholesterol deposits).

We measured these fractions in our first niacin study and found that the drug (not a vitamin at these doses) reduced the bad cholesterol and increased the good fraction. These are desirable changes, not matched even today by any other cholesterol control drug. Any doctors who think the significance of LDL and HDL cholesterol fractions was first discovered during the 1970's may be surprised to learn that the fractions were known and favorably altered by niacin in this 1955-1956 study.

Before leaving Rochester in April 1956 to practice with a multispecialty clinic in Madison, Wisconsin, I presented the results of this work at a Mayo Clinic staff meeting. The paper was published later that spring in the *Proceedings of the Staff Meetings of the Mayo Clinic*, the widely circulated journal which since then has shortened its name to *Mayo Clinic Proceedings*. In November 1956 I first reported our results, updated somewhat by further follow-up, at a national meeting. This was the annual fall meeting in Chicago of the American Society for the Study of Arteriosclerosis (later to become the Council on Arteriosclerosis of the American Heart Association), a group to which I would then report further studies of niacin every year through 1972.

As I continued to study the new method of treatment in Madison, my Mayo colleagues extended the study we had started there. Meanwhile, others around the world learned of niacin's success and included it in their own clinical investigations. Most of what we know about how to handle niacin was learned and reported in the first five years after its introduction, much of it in my writings and those of the Mayo group. It is difficult for doctors to locate those reports today since computer searches ordinarily cover only the past ten years. My chapters in two books, Rudolf Altschul's *Niacin in Vascular Disorders and Hyperlipemia* (1964), or Dick Casdorph's *Treatment of the Hyperlipidemic States* (1971), contain useful bibliographies of the early publications, as do other chapters in the Altschul work.

By 1963, National Institutes of Health (NIH) recognized that it was better to have a lower rather than a higher cholesterol level. This led them to pose the question of whether any drugs were ready for study in a large field trial to determine whether cholesterol control reduced coronary disease and other cholesterol deposits in arteries (atherosclerosis). Ken Berge and I served on the *ad hoc* committee assembled to address this question. (Sadly, our dear friend and colleague, Dick Achor, had died of acute leukemia in 1962.) We decided that several drugs were "ready" and began the planning which led to the Coronary Drug Project (1966-1974), the first nationwide multicenter study of any kind. This study and its important findings were mentioned briefly in the Introduction to this book. The CDP was the first study to demonstrate that a drug to reduce blood lipids (fat-like substances) would lessen heart attacks, strokes, and cardiovascular surgery. Of the several drugs studied, only niacin produced these benefits. Then, in a survey several years later, an average of fifteen years after enrollment, niacin proved to be the only drug in the study to reduce total deaths as well.

Since its earliest use as the first cholesterol-control agent, niacin has been a generic drug. Because no company can hold a patent and reap large profits from its exclusive sale, niacin has never had a huge advertising campaign or a flock of sales representatives to announce its successes to physicians, as have the newer, expensive drugs. In recent years, many studies have been funded by companies which market competing drugs and often show this bias, even in the few studies that combined niacin with other cholesterol-control agents. Since some of their studies are funded and their travels subsidized by the manufacturers of expensive drugs, well-known spokesmen in the field of lipid metabolism are not likely to point out niacin's distinctive advantages on all the lipid fractions, on cardiovascular events, and on the patient's pocketbook.

When pharmaceutical representatives touting other drugs (or other niacin detractors) label niacin as "hard to take," with "side effects and toxic effects," who can blame the average practitioner for selecting another drug for cholesterol control? Because resins are more intolerable to patients than niacin has ever been, clinicians often turn to the coenzyme A reductase inhibitors (sometimes shortened to "co-A reductase inhibitors," or simply "statins"). This group now includes lovastatin (Mevacor), pravastatin, (Pravachol), simvastatin (Zocor), fluvastatin (Lescol), atorvastatin (Lipitor) and probably will include other statins yet to come.

A decision to use these drugs ignores the fact that the statins have not been on the market nearly as long as niacin, and new adverse effects are still being discovered. It also ignores the well-known possibilities of liver damage from use of statins, as well as muscular problems. These include muscle pains, tenderness, abnormal muscle enzymes in the blood, or even destruction of muscle fibers. A later chapter reviews this drug group and others in more detail, spelling out a new danger, first reported early in 1997 and not known to most doctors at this writing.

Finally, a decision to use one of the "statins" overlooks the major consideration of lifetime expense if one spends from $65 to $210 a month for Mevacor vs. eight to ten dollars a month for niacin. (These figures, here and throughout the book, are based on our 1997 survey in Scottsdale, Arizona pharmacies.) Translated into $780 to $2,520 annually for Mevacor and $96 to $120 for niacin, the difference is even more impressive. If projected to the millions of American adults with cholesterol patterns that make them candidates for treatment, according to NCEP guidelines, the differences in annual expenditures on drugs for cholesterol control in U.S. would amount to billions of dollars.

Remember: Although available over-the-counter, without prescription, *niacin is not a do-it-yourself drug!* It needs to be taken under *knowledgeable medical supervision.* In other words, it should not only be supervised by a doctor but by one who knows what he is doing. Your physician should be *"good at niacin."*

By becoming adept in using niacin, a doctor can treat his patients with an agent that reduces cardiovascular complications and their expensive, life-altering accompaniments (coronary bypass surgery, angioplasty, atherectomy, stents, and the like). This skill can allow a patient to avoid living the rest of his life as a heart attack survivor. Instead he can enjoy life as one who has not had a heart attack. To the physician, this should be a source of great satisfaction; to the patient, it should be an incentive to find a doctor who is good at niacin.

CHAPTER TWO

Why Is It Important to Control Cholesterol?

Cardiovascular Disease: What Are We Up Against?

Cardiovascular diseases remain the leading cause of death in the United States and all developed countries of the world. Most deaths are caused by heart attacks and strokes, which also cause much long-term disability in the aging population. Atherosclerosis, the process by which cholesterol plaques lead to narrowing of arteries and their eventual occlusion, is responsible for nearly all this cardiovascular disease, death, and disability.

The number of Americans killed in World War I, World War II, the Korean conflict, and Vietnam is given as 425,974. The number of deaths in the United States from cardiovascular disease in 1990 was estimated at 930,477. Besides deaths and reduction in quality of life for victims of heart attacks and strokes, the cost of caring for these patients is the largest part of the American health care budget. Unquestionably, atherosclerotic disease should be prevented, to the extent that this is possible.

About one-third of persons die of the first heart attack. *In many individuals, the first manifestation of coronary disease is sudden death!* If we were to wait for symptoms, we would have no chance to help this large number of persons. To reduce this devastating toll, researchers for several decades have studied *risk factors* which foretell the development of atherosclerosis in the coronary arteries and throughout the body. Although called *coronary* risk factors, they also apply to atherosclerotic deposits in other areas.

Coronary Risk Factors

Many studies, notably the Framingham (Massachusetts) Study, performed for several decades under National Institutes of Health (NIH) auspices, have identified a number of factors, that predict the development of atherosclerotic disease. Some factors cannot be altered: *age*, *sex*, and *strong family history of coronary disease*. Formerly only *male sex* was listed among the risk factors; recent guidelines have changed this to *male or postmenopausal female*. Although one's heredity cannot be changed, a strong family history should lead a person to do everything he/she can do to normalize risk factors which can be measured and, if abnormal, improved. If a close male relative has had a heart attack or stroke *before age 50* or a female relative *before age 60*, you have a significant family history. All adults, not just those with a family history, should know their risk factors and improve any that are abnormal.

The major risk factors that can be corrected if abnormal are *smoking, hypertension* (high blood pressure), *abnormal cholesterol levels*, *diabetes, physical inactivity*, and *obesity*. Of these, the first three (smoking, hypertension, and abnormal cholesterol levels) are the most significant. Treatment of these factors has the greatest effect in reducing the morbidity (illness and disability) and mortality (deaths) from artery-narrowing disorders.

Reduction in cigarette smoking and effective control of blood pressure by excellent drugs have reduced heart attacks and strokes. Smoking a pack of cigarettes daily doubles the risk of heart attack or stroke, but stopping smoking eliminates this excessive risk in a relatively short time. It does not remove the risks of lung cancer or emphysema, which are related to total lifetime exposure to inhaled smoke; however, by quitting, one stops adding to these risks. At one time, studies appeared to indicate that proper control of high blood pressure reduced the risk of stroke but not of heart attack. Recent work shows that heart attacks are also reduced, which makes more sense.

I remember well an evening in the late 1960's when I was working with a colleague in Madison on data from our clinical studies with drugs to reduce high blood pressure. In discussing coronary risk factors, we agreed that *the day would come when a heart attack would be considered a therapeutic failure.*

In 1994 William B. Kannel, M.D. received the highest scientific honor of the American Heart Association (AHA), its Research Achievement Award. This honor was based on Dr. Kannel's accomplishments as long-time medical director of the Framingham Heart Study, which taught us most of what we know today about coronary risk factors. His acceptance speech included this sentence: "The day must come when we consider a heart attack in our patients not as the first indication for treatment but as a medical failure." This took me back to that evening in the 1960's when my colleague and I had predicted that this would come to pass. We should, now or in the near future, consider each heart attack a medical failure, either attributed to the patient's negligence in taking care of himself and obtaining proper preventive care, or the doctor's failure to provide that care.

Who Needs Cholesterol Control?

How many Americans need treatment for cholesterol abnormalities? I posed this question to James Cleeman, M.D., coordinator of the National Cholesterol Education Program (NCEP) at National Institutes of Health (NIH). What were his best estimates of the numbers of American adults who have cholesterol levels or fractions ("bad" and "good" cholesterol) which make them candidates for treatment, according to the 1993 NCEP guidelines? He replied *52 million (about 29% of adults)*. He added that about 12 to 13 million adults have coronary disease. *Almost all of them* need drug therapy to reach the current goals, and only 25% to 30% of them are receiving *any* treatment. These figures are based on the third National Health and Nutrition Examination Survey (NHANES III) and the 1993 NCEP guidelines. However, the figures address only total cholesterol, except in persons with coronary disease, and do not address the "good" cholesterol levels at all. In truth, the numbers in need of cholesterol control are higher, probably much higher.

In 1994 coronary heart disease was responsible for the deaths of about 500,000 Americans, while stroke killed more than 140,000. Cardiovascular disease claims an American life every 34 seconds. In patients under 50, cigarettes are related to 80% of cardiovascular deaths. American Heart Association (AHA) has projected that cessation of smoking alone could reduce mortality by 40%. In 1995, AHA estimated that only one-fifth to one-third of patients with coronary events who are candidates for secondary prevention measures (preventive treatment after such an event) are receiving them—and the situation has not improved since then.

Suffice it to say that a very large number of American adults need cholesterol control, probably exceeding the 29% quoted by NCEP. As we consider this situation further, you will see where you and others close to you stand in this regard. You will learn that diet is a weak and often ineffective method of changing cholesterol and why niacin, from the available drugs, should be the first choice. This ideal drug could be the eventual treatment for 90% or more of those needing cholesterol control—if all doctors were good at niacin.

"Bad" and "Good" Cholesterol

In earlier years, most observers considered only the *total* cholesterol level when assessing coronary risk factors. As time went on, the importance of controlling both the low-density lipoprotein (LDL) cholesterol, the *"bad"* cholesterol fraction, and the high-density lipoprotein (HDL) cholesterol, the *"good"* cholesterol fraction, became apparent.

The significance of the "bad" and "good" cholesterol fractions was actually known and their measurements included in my pioneer report on niacin's use to reduce cholesterol in 1956, as well as in all my subsequent papers about work in this field. However, the "establishment" re-discovered and re-named these fractions in the 1970's. In 1993, NIH's National Cholesterol Education Program (NCEP) "Expert Panel" recommended specific goals for treatment of both LDL and HDL fractions.

What makes LDL cholesterol (LDLC) bad and HDL cholesterol (HDLC) good? LDLC is deposited in plaques in the walls of arteries, resulting in narrowing and eventual blockage in some instances. HDLC, on the other hand, is not deposited and has a protective action by "unloading" cholesterol deposits from arterial plaques. Figure 1 depicts these characteristics in cartoon fashion, which you will remember after you forget my words.

How to remember which is which, good or bad? Just remember that "H" stands for *healthy* and "L" stands for *lousy*. This memory device is not elegant, but it works.

National Cholesterol Education Program (NCEP) Guidelines

The "Expert Panel" of the National Cholesterol Education Program (NCEP) of National Institutes of Health (NIH) issued its first set of guidelines for diagnosis and treatment of cholesterol problems in 1988. (I choose to put "Expert Panel" in quotes because I feel that the group does not show much expertise in use of niacin or recognize its distinctive advantages, as detailed in this book. Its guidelines do not even spell out the important differences

Figure 1

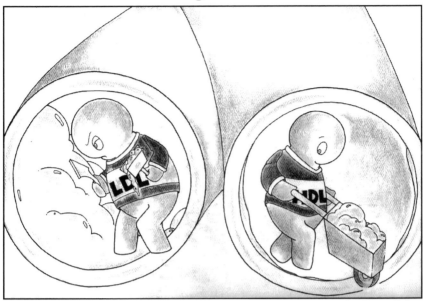

LDL ("bad") cholesterol is like a plasterer, heaping plaques onto the inner lining of arteries. HDL ("good") cholesterol works in the opposite direction "unloading" cholesterol from arterial plaques.

How to remember which is which? H stands for healthy; L stands for lousy. This memory device is not elegant, but it works.

between plain niacin and time-release niacin, which both patient and physician need to know.)

The NCEP Panel's second report, in 1993, contained several refinements. The list of risk factors was changed slightly. Instead of just male sex, they added postmenopausal status in women as a risk factor. They also added family history of a premature heart attack or sudden death (before age 50 in male, before age 60 in female).

HDL (good) cholesterol had been largely ignored in the 1988 guidelines. The 1993 guidelines recommended treating HDL cholesterol if *below 35*[1] since HDL cholesterol below this level is the only abnormal risk factor which can be identified in a fair number of persons who have heart attacks. But what is the target level for treatment? NCEP doesn't say.

---

[1] Other countries, notably Canada, use a different numerical system to designate cholesterol values. The *Systeme Internationale* uses SI units rather than the metric system traditionally used in the U.S. over the years. (Most, but not all, U.S. medical journals now express laboratory values in both ways. I will add a further brief comment in the Medical Section.) Appendix B is a table showing how to convert mg% values to SI units.

19

Obviously we can't just get the HDLC fraction to 36, heave a sigh of relief and decide we are out of trouble, because we're not. We need a cushion above the 35 borderline. I like to see the HDLC level at 45 or higher. Such levels are usually not difficult to achieve with niacin.

If HDLC is *high* (above 60), the guidelines *subtract* one risk factor, based on the protective action of HDLC. This is important to remember as we consider treatment with niacin, which often raises HDLC above this level.

In 1993 NCEP also defined several target levels for LDL (bad) cholesterol, based on the number of abnormal risk factors or the presence of clinical atherosclerotic disease. They advised bringing the LDLC level to *100 or less* in anyone who has had a heart attack, chest pain from coronary disease, previous coronary artery surgery, angioplasty, or any of the newer procedures for widening narrowed arteries. This guideline (LDLC 100 or less) also applies to persons with a previous stroke due to a blood clot or those with narrowing, blockage, or surgery of neck or leg arteries. For other persons, NCEP advises LDLC *below 130* if there are *two or more* risk factors. NCEP called a level of LDLC *below 160* satisfactory if *fewer than two* risk factors are present, but *I prefer to see LDLC below 130 in everyone.*

Some physicians like to use the *ratio* of total cholesterol to HDLC (TC/HDLC ratio) to predict likelihood of coronary disease and to decide on treatment options. Some observers have reported that this ratio is a better predictor than single numbers: total cholesterol (TC), LDLC, or HDLC. This may be so, but when treating a patient, I prefer not to use the ratio, since it is based on two numbers and therefore influenced by variations in either TC or HDLC. Instead, I look at LDLC and HDLC fractions singly. If both are in proper ranges, *it really doesn't matter what the total cholesterol is!* This is ironic, because for years the NCEP (and doctors who cared about their patients) tried to get patients to know that "cholesterol number"" and try to keep it in the desirable range. Now it turns out that the total cholesterol "number," while a general guide, can be deceptive.

Here are a couple of examples which illustrate this point. A man has a total cholesterol level of 182, in the below-200 "desirable" range. His LDL (bad) cholesterol fraction also looks good at 130. However, his HDL (good) fraction is only 30, in the dangerous below-35 range. The sum of LDLC plus HDLC does not equal the TC because there's one more fraction, which we don't talk about much, the *very low-density lipoprotein (VLDL) cholesterol*, which usually runs between 15 and 25—in this hypothetical case, 22.

Table 1

	"Desirable"	Example 1	Example 2
Total cholesterol (TC)	200 or less	182	245
Low density lipoprotein cholesterol (LDLC)	Varies*	130	145
High density lipoprotein cholesterol (HDLC)	45 or higher	30	80
Very low density lipo-protein cholesterol (VLDLC)	No standard	22	20

Two examples (see text) of how total cholesterol can be misleading if both LDLC and HDLC are not measured. Example 1, with TC in the "desirable" range, shows a dangerously low HDLC level. Example 2, with TC in a "too high" range, has satisfactory LDLC and very high HDLC; the latter can be achieved by estrogen replacement in postmenopausal women—or by niacin.

> * NCEP accepts LDLC below 160 if fewer than two risk factors or below 130 if two or more risk factors with no demonstrated vascular disease but advises LDLC below 100 if one has had a cardiovascular event or significant atherosclerotic lesion.

Or consider the postmenopausal woman with no other risk factors and total cholesterol of 245—higher than the "desirable" 200. Her LDLC is 145, low enough to satisfy NCEP guidelines (below 160 if only one risk factor). However, she is taking estrogens and her HDLC is 80! The VLDLC of 20 makes up the difference. Table 1 shows the cholesterol fractions in these two hypothetical patients, showing that total cholesterol is really irrelevant and can be misleading unless you know what the bad and good cholesterol fractions are.

Diet for Cholesterol Control

Although recommended by diet advocates, including the NCEP, *diet is a weak and often ineffective means of controlling cholesterol*. A 1993 book on this subject, *Coronary Heart Disease: The Dietary Sense and Nonsense*[2], contains a critical review of medical literature concerned with diet, cholesterol, heart disease, and death. This multi-author book concludes that *diet is not effective* in control of cholesterol, reducing it only during periods of

---

[2] When quoting from this book, I may simply call it "George Mann's book" or just "Mann's book." He not only edited the book but also organized the symposium on which it was based.

weight loss. My experience agrees with the viewpoint of this book, which will be discussed in Chapter 4, *Why Not Diet To Control Cholesterol?*

In this regard, a notable NIH-sponsored study of the early 1960's, the Diet-Heart Feasibility Trial (1963-1965), showed that most people would not follow diets with significant limitation of fat and cholesterol; furthermore, it didn't make much difference if they did. As my chapter in the above-mentioned book pointed out, "The study had carefully chosen clinical centers, highly motivated and carefully educated patients, strong dietetic support, expensive food distribution centers, and specially prepared foods not then (or now) generally available, and still it failed." Despite poor adherence and lack of efficacy, those who performed the study declared the Diet-Heart Feasibility Trial a success and recommended that a massive national study be undertaken without delay. This suggestion was rejected, avoiding the expenditure of vast amounts of money and human energy on a project which clearly would have been doomed to fail.

The Coronary Drug Project

During the same years another NIH-sponsored group planned a long-term multicenter trial of cholesterol-altering drugs and coronary disease, the Coronary Drug Project (CDP), mentioned earlier. In 1966 the CDP began enrolling about 7,700 men, ages 30 to 65, who had already had one or more heart attacks. They randomly assigned these participants to a drug or placebo in groups matched in regard to known coronary risk factors. The drugs were niacin, clofibrate (Atromid-S), d-thyroxine (Choloxin), and two dosage levels of a female hormone (Premarin). Major endpoints were death, proven heart attack, stroke or related event; other important observations included hospitalization from all causes, cardiovascular hospitalization, and cardiovascular surgery.

A total of 53 medical centers from Massachusetts to Hawaii required about three years to recruit 7,700 participants. They then followed each man for at least five years, so the entire study continued until 1974. The CDP followed some of its earlier enrollees for more than eight years.

D-thyroxine was dropped early in the study when it was found to be causing more heart attacks than the placebo. Next, the two dosage levels of Premarin (2.5 mg per day and 1.25 mg per day) showed more clotting problems, including heart attacks, so they too were dropped.

Niacin (then usually called *nicotinic acid*[3] in this country) and clofibrate were the only drugs to finish the study, with at least five years of treatment for each participant. Clofibrate showed no beneficial effect on cardiovascular endpoints and was associated with troublesome problems, including an increase in gallstones. Niacin, on the other hand, reduced nonfatal heart attacks, strokes and related events, cardiovascular surgery, cardiovascular hospitalization, and all hospitalization—the only drug to show any of these benefits. Table 2 compares the effects of niacin and placebo on CDP endpoints. Niacin reduced both nonfatal heart attacks (myocardial infarctions) and strokes or related events by about 25% while cutting the need for cardiovascular surgery nearly in half (46% reduction).

When death rates were compared immediately after the study, there was a trend toward a reduced mortality rate in men receiving niacin for longer than five years, but it was not statistically significant. For nine years after the end of the CDP, niacin detractors repeatedly contended that its success in the CDP was, after all, not significant since total deaths had not been reduced!

Nine years after the CDP ended, its statisticians surveyed the 53 centers to determine how many participants were still alive and how many had died. Remember that each participant had suffered one or more heart attacks before enrolling in the CDP at ages 30 to 65, which means that some had reached age 80 by this time. When this survey was done, average time since enrollment was fifteen years.

Table 3 compares the effects of niacin and placebo on deaths from all causes in CDP participants, as reported in the 15-year survey. In the placebo group, the percentage of men who had died from all causes was 58.2%. For all drug groups except niacin, total deaths were in the same range as placebo, 57% to 59%. In the niacin group, only 52.0% had died. The statisticians calculated that the difference between placebo and niacin (58.2% vs. 52.0%) represents *11% fewer deaths* in the niacin group. Looking at the figures another way, median survival time from entry into the study was 11.40 years

---

[3] The change in designation (from *nicotinic acid* to *niacin*) has been gradual over the years. It has also been incomplete; occasionally an author will still use "nicotinic acid" in current writing. I do not know exactly the reason or the dynamics of the change in terminology, but I have welcomed it. In the early days the similarity between "nicotinic acid" and "nicotine" caused a certain amount of confusion among patients, leading some to ask, "Oh, that means I should smoke more to lower my cholesterol?" *Niacin* is shorter, crisper, and a name known to most people who have ever seen ads for foods containing the vitamin. Now we just have to cope with the thought process that niacin is "only a vitamin" and, by implication, a harmless agent to take. Hence my frequent warning: When used for cholesterol control, niacin is *not* a vitamin. It is a *drug* with decidedly favorable effects when used under skilled medical supervision but with potential for harm if misused or taken without such supervision.

for placebo, compared with 13.03 years for the niacin group. *Niacin added an average of 1.63 years of life* in these heart attack survivors.

These strikingly successful results are even more remarkable when one considers how the CDP protocol was biased (unintentionally, I think) against cholesterol-lowering drugs, particularly niacin. The participants were chosen, not by cholesterol levels but because of previous heart attacks. As a result, about 50% had cholesterol levels lower than 250 (then considered normal) at entry. If all men had had high cholesterol levels, even more difference between placebo and niacin would have been likely, both in cholesterol levels and in events, including deaths.

The maximum daily dose of niacin in the CDP was 3.0 grams (g) per day. A fixed dose might have been suitable for the other study drugs, but in actual practice the dose of niacin needs to be adjusted according to each patient's response. Since many patients need larger doses to provide better cholesterol control, the results of niacin therapy in medical practice should actually exceed those of the CDP. It's too bad the daily dose of niacin in the CDP was not 4.5 g, which also would have improved the results. In the early years we customarily started with 3.0 g per day, but at least 50% of patients in my studies needed a larger dose, 4.5 g or 6.0 g.

Table 2
Comparison of Niacin and Placebo
in Major Cardiovascular Events:
Coronary Drug Project (1966-1974)

	Placebo	Niacin	Difference
Nonfatal myocardial infarction	12.2%	8.9%	-27%
Strokes & transient ischemic attacks	11.2%	8.5%	-24%
Hospitalized for cardiovascular disease	32.4%	28.5%	-12%
Cardiovascular surgery	4.9%	2.6%	-46%

Note that nonfatal heart attacks as well as strokes and related events were each reduced by about one-fourth in participants receiving niacin. Cardiovascular surgery was reduced by nearly one-half.

Table 3
Comparison in Total Deaths (All Causes),
Niacin vs. Placebo
(Follow-Up Survey, Coronary Drug Project)

	Placebo	Niacin	Difference
Death from all causes	58.2%	52.0%	-11%
Median survival time from entry (years)	11.40	13.03	+1.63

Mean follow-up time was 15 years after enrollment in the study. At entry each participant was between 30 and 65 years of age, with one or more previous heart attacks. The difference in rates of deaths from all causes is highly significant (p=0.0004). See text for further discussion.

Until the CDP, we early workers with niacin had to be careful to say that we could not be sure that the favorable lipid changes would result in reduction of atherosclerotic disease (arterial narrowing by cholesterol plaques). Remember the classic kindergarten experiment in which a rat fed proper foods thrived and had a beautiful coat while another rat fed only candy and snacks became malnourished and its hair fell out? When the teacher asked a little boy what he learned from the experiment, he replied that a rat shouldn't eat only candy and snacks. This boy did not take his conclusions beyond the scope of his data. That's the way we had to hedge until the results of the CDP showed that niacin *did* reduce clinical events and deaths—the first such demonstration for any drug.

How could taking niacin for five to eight years have reduced deaths in the 15-year survey? Two explanations are possible; it is likely that both contributed to the favorable outcome. They are (1) regression of plaques in arteries and (2) stabilization of plaques likely to rupture.

Regression Studies

The term *regression studies* refers to trials which have shown not only retardation of new cholesterol deposits in walls of arteries but also reduction of some existing plaques. Persons with recent coronary arteriograms (artery x-rays), performed for clinical reasons, have enrolled in controlled studies to compare an active form of cholesterol control with placebo. Usually investigators have repeated artery x-rays after two years; one study also rechecked them after four years. Observers then compared the arteriograms

25

without knowing which patients had received active drugs or other treatment and which did not. For that matter, they did not know whether x-rays of each arterial segment were presented in the "before-after" or "after-before" sequence.

Measuring the diameters of coronary arteries at places narrowed by atherosclerotic plaques, these studies detected whether previous cholesterol deposits improved or became worse. Various groups studied several drugs, singly or in combination. In most studies, reducing total and LDL (bad) cholesterol resulted in retardation of new deposits and some regression in older deposits. Experts in flow of liquids tell us that even very small increases in arterial diameter can improve blood flow considerably.

Regression of cholesterol plaques in CDP participants taking niacin, could explain, at least in part, reduction in the overall death rate in the follow-up survey years later. Because aggressively reducing total and LDL cholesterol led to regression of arterial plaques, regardless of the method used, the 1993 NCEP Panel recommended that LDL cholesterol be reduced to less than 100 in persons with proven atherosclerotic disease. Regression occurs in other locations as well, of course, not just in coronary arteries.

At least ten studies have been done, using different methods of treatment. Each led to regression of plaques, demonstrating one mechanism by which cholesterol control can reduce heart attacks and other atherosclerotic events. However, as time passed, observers pointed out that the changes in arterial diameter were quite small. To explain the observed improvement in clinical endpoints, one would have to invoke the pronouncement of the flow experts that even small increases in diameter result in considerable enhancement of blood flow. Or there may be a more plausible mechanism by which drugs can prevent arterial blockage and save lives. These two mechanisms probably work together.

Prevention of Plaque Rupture

In the past few years a second mechanism has intrigued experts, who are still studying it. Sometimes a plaque narrowing an artery by only 50% (not much, in terms of the 80% to 90% narrowing which leads to surgery or other intervention) *ruptures*, leading to immediate occlusion of the artery. Drugs for cholesterol control tend to *stabilize these rupture-prone plaques*, making such an event less likely.

A rupture-prone plaque is like a volcano getting ready to erupt. Its center (lava in the volcano) is made up of "foam cells," rich in lipids.[4] A weak fibrous cap covers this pool of lipids. Cholesterol-regulating therapy stabilizes rupture-prone plaques in several ways. These include depleting the lipid pool and normalizing function of the arterial lining covering the plaque, as well as other mechanisms. Interestingly, Rudolf Altschul (one of the Canadians who, in 1955, first suggested that niacin reduced cholesterol) reported in 1957 that niacin reduced the lipid content of foam cells in the arterial linings of cholesterol-fed rabbits. This is one of the ways that cholesterol control drugs can stabilize rupture-prone plaques.

Experts have decided that plaque rupture underlies many cardiac events, which are mainly determined by the composition of plaques, not the degree of narrowing. There is no connective tissue at the surface of the cap over the lipid core. If a fissure forms in the cap, blood seeps in from the bloodstream and leads to formation of a clot, which can block the artery, leading to a heart attack or other clinical event. Lipid-controlling drugs stabilize the rupture-prone plaque, thus preventing this occlusion.

Niacin's Distinctive Advantages

In the 1988 guidelines and again in 1993, NCEP designated niacin and a pair of agents called *bile-sequestrant resins* (cholestyramine and colestipol) as the "first-line" drugs for cholesterol control, based on their long safety records and their demonstrated ability to reduce heart attacks and deaths, as well as controlling cholesterol. Mann's book explains in some detail why the reduction in heart attacks and deaths by cholestyramine resin (Questran) in the major research trial of this drug is questionable. I will review this in Chapter 8, *The Other Drugs for Cholesterol Control*. In 1993, NCEP added to the list of "major drugs" a group of agents nicknamed "statins," since each of their generic names ends in those two syllables.

NCEP should recognize that niacin is the ideal drug for control of cholesterol and its fractions. It reduces total cholesterol and low-density lipoprotein (LDL, "bad") cholesterol, increases high-density lipoprotein (HDL, "good") cholesterol, and reduces triglycerides. Niacin is the only drug with all these favorable characteristics. Table 4 shows its superiority,

---

[4] *Lipids* are fat-like substances, the most familiar of which are cholesterol and triglycerides. They circulate in the blood attached to proteins (lipoproteins) of several sizes and densities, which partly determine whether they will be included in artery-narrowing plaques or play a role in reducing these deposits.

comparing current drugs for cholesterol control by showing which goals of treatment they achieve. The *bile-sequestering resins*, long the favorites of NIH for reasons best known to their leaders, do not reduce HDLC or triglycerides. Neither do the *"statins,"* the largest-selling drugs for cholesterol control, in spite of their high costs, which result from expensive promotions in TV, newspaper, and magazine ads, plus a sales force visiting doctors nationwide. The *fibrates* (only one in the U.S., gemfibrozil) do nothing for LDLC and TC. In my experience they are also disappointing in raising low HDLC, and FDA recommends limiting their use. (See Chapter 8, *The Other Drugs for Cholesterol Control.*) Finally, these other drugs have not been reported to be effective without dietary limitation, as niacin has.

Table 4
Are goals of lipid control met by various drugs?

	Total & LDLC	HDLC	Tri- glycerides	Without Diet
Niacin	+	+	+	+
Resins	+	0	0	0
Statins	+	0	0*	0
Fibrates	0	+	+	0

(+ = can achieve this goal; 0 = does not)

Resins: cholestyramine (Questran), colestipol (Colestid)

Statins: lovastatin (Mevacor), simvastatin (Zocor), pravastatin (Pravachol), fluvastatin (Lescol), atorvastatin (Lipitor)

Fibrates: gemfibrozil

*Atorvastatin, introduced in 1997, is the only statin which reduces triglycerides.

Niacin is the only cholesterol-control drug shown to reduce heart attacks, strokes and related events, cardiovascular surgery, cardiovascular hospitalization, and all hospitalization, as well as total deaths. No other drug has all of these distinctive advantages or niacin's long safety record, dating to 1955. Table 5 compares the effects of major cholesterol drugs on these clinical endpoints. Whether a resin actually reduced heart attacks and strokes in the only large trial of its effect is open to question, as explained in Chapter 8. That chapter also mentions recent studies in Scandinavia and Scotland, which did show reduction in heart attacks and deaths with two of the "statins."

The single large trial of the fibrate, gemfibrozil, performed in Finland, found reduction in heart attacks but none of the other clinical benefits.

Sometimes some one asks, "What's new about a cholesterol-control drug that has been around for 40 years?" There are several answers. Listing niacin's superior spectrum of lipid and clinical effects, just reviewed, should be enough. But there's more. Every time there is a new discovery in cholesterol metabolism with an influence on coronary risk, investigators study the effect of existing treatments. Each time, the outcome has been *more good news about niacin!* And in each instance, with one exception, all the other drugs have failed to help.

Table 5
Are clinical goals of cholesterol control met by various drugs?

	MI	Stroke or TIA	CV Surg	CV Hosp	All Hosp	Death
Niacin	+	+	+	+	+	+
Resins	?	0	0	0	0	??
Statins	+	+	+	–	--	+
Fibrates	+	0	0	0	0	0

(+ = can achieve this goal; 0 = does not; – = not reported)

Resins: cholestyramine (Questran), colestipol (Colestid)

Statins: lovastatin (Mevacor), simvastatin (Zocor), pravastatin (Pravachol), fluvastatin (Lescol), atorvastatin (Lipitor)

Fibrates: gemfibrozil (Lopid)

MI = myocardial infarction (heart attack)
TIA = transient ischemic attack (stroke warning)
CV = cardiovascular (surgery/hospitalization)

These have been the new research discoveries in recent years which are all favorably altered by niacin but by no other cholesterol-control drugs:

- Niacin reduces *lipoprotein (a)*, abbreviated *Lp(a)*, pronounced "LP little A." This special form of LDL cholesterol has been found to be a strong predictor of heart attack and stroke.

29

- When niacin raises HDLC, practically all of the increase is in the most protective subfraction, HDL_2. This increases the ratio of HDL_2 to HDL_3, a favorable change.

- Niacin also converts small-particle LDLC to large-particle, another change calculated to reduce risk.

With one exception, niacin is the *only* agent that accomplishes *any* of these desirable effects. The exception: estrogens (female hormones), given to postmenopausal women, can reduce Lp(a). The above-listed accomplishments add to niacin's distinctive advantages, all of them reasons to choose niacin as the *only* drug of first choice. These three measurements are research procedures, not performed routinely in clinical practice of medicine. But this doesn't matter. A doctor planning treatment for his patients *knows* that these favorable changes occur with niacin but with *no other drug*.

We must remember that niacin's low cost is one of its distinctive advantages. It is the only inexpensive drug for cholesterol control, by a large margin. Table 6 compares these costs. The figures speak for themselves.

According to a recent estimate, about two-thirds of Americans have pharmacy plans that allow them to obtain medications for a nominal co-payment, so you may be saying that the decided cost advantage of niacin doesn't really matter to you. Furthermore, some plans do not pay for over-the-counter drugs (aspirin, Tylenol, antacids, etc.). Using this as a reason, some plans fail to include niacin in their formularies; others include only plain niacin, based on the mistaken belief that time-release niacin should be avoided. You need to know that for eight to ten dollars a month (about the same as your co-payment for the expensive drugs) you can use by far the best treatment for cholesterol control. Remember, some one is paying high prices for those expensive drugs that do not accomplish all of niacin's benefits, whether it is the pharmacy plan or HMO ("health maintenance organization"). Ultimately you are the one who pays.

Brainwashing the Public and the Medical Profession

Why, then, have dietary advocates kept insisting that diet should be the first and foremost method of treatment for cholesterol abnormalities? In George Mann's book, he speculates on possible reasons. George believes that American Heart Association (AHA) clings to its diet advocacy because its fund-raising program would collapse if the organization admitted that diet, always a cornerstone of its recommendations to the public, is ineffective.

Likewise, he states that the National Heart, Lung, and Blood Institute (NHLBI) at NIH cannot admit to Congress that it has wasted billions of dollars in support of diet-related research. He also blames the food industry, which has a huge investment in advertising foods as low in cholesterol, "heart-smart" or just plain "healthy," even though no evidence exists that any type of dietary manipulation prevents heart attacks or reduces total deaths.

Over the years, opinion-making and policy-making bodies at AHA, NIH, and elsewhere have been dominated by investigators whose careers

Table 6
Costs of Cholesterol-Control Drugs

	Daily Dose	Monthly Cost
Niacin		
Time-Release (Endur-acin)	1.5 g/day	$8
	2.0 g/day	$10
Plain	3.0 g/day	$6.50
	4.5 g/day	$9.75
	6.0 g/day	$13.50
Bile-Sequestrant Resins		
Cholestyramine (Questran)	12 g/day	$86
	16 g/day	$115
	24 g/day	$172
Colestipol (Colestid)	15 g/day	$74
	20 g/day	$99
	30 g/day	$148
HMG CoA Reductase Inhibitors		
Lovastatin (Mevacor)	20 mg/day	$55
	40 mg/day	$105
	80 mg/day	$210

Table 6 (continued)		
HMG CoA Reductase Inhibitors (continued)		
Pravastatin (Pravachol)	10 mg/day	$48
	20 mg/day	$52
	40 mg/day	$92
Simvastatin (Zocor)	5 mg/day	$51
	10 mg/day	$56
	20 mg/day	$97
	40 mg/day	$102
Fluvastatin (Lescol)	20 mg/day	$34
	40 mg/day	$37
Atorvastatin (Lipitor)	10 mg/day	$55
	20 mg/day	$84
	40 mg/day	$111
	80 mg/day	$222
Fibrates		
Gemfibrozil (Lopid)	1200 mg/day	$73
(generic)	1200 mg/day	$30

were devoted to research associated with diet. Their advocacy of diet as the major method for cholesterol control permeated many scientific organizations and flooded the medical literature over the years. A second generation of diet advocates succeeded the first—a self-perpetuating dynasty. It is amazing that the medical profession accepted their preachings for so long with blind faith. This has begun to change in recent years, but the domination of believers in the diet-heart myth has not yet been overcome. These opinion-makers have brainwashed the media, which in turn has brainwashed the public, including the medical profession.

How can the medical profession be deluded, along with the public? The average physician, burdened with the impossible task of trying to keep up in many facets of medicine, does not read critically all that is published about cholesterol control. He finds it comfortable, therefore, to accept the pronouncements of "experts" and published "guidelines."

Until recently the "experts" have held out for diet as primary treatment for abnormal cholesterol values. Fortunately, the pendulum has swung away from using diet for six months (the 1988 NCEP guidelines) to unspecified shorter periods, with earlier use of medications when diet fails. Over the years, many clinicians have recognized in their own practices the futility of diet for cholesterol control and have moved sooner to effective treatment with medication.

To get a divergent viewpoint into the media is still difficult, almost impossible. Typically, a writer or producer calls the local Heart Association or one of its physicians to ask about the dissenting opinion. The spokesperson parrots the party line about diet. The writer or producer believes this dogma since it agrees with what he has heard all along. Thus the public, including the medical profession, is brainwashed further when the opposing view (which happens to be correct) is not published or aired.

Not only did the 1988 NCEP guidelines recommend a six-month trial of diet before considering drug treatment; the "Expert Panel" advised starting with the AHA "Step One" diet, then *making the diet stricter* if cholesterol goals were not reached by the end of three months. They seemed to forget, if they had ever known, the lessons of the Diet-Heart Feasibility Trial of the early 1960's: People will not follow diets designed to control cholesterol, and it doesn't make much difference if they do.

Apparently they were also unfamiliar with (or chose to ignore) the dozens of reports in the late 1950's and 1960's that niacin's favorable effects on blood cholesterol occur *without alteration of the usual American diet.* Finally, the "experts," most of them academicians or researchers, not practicing physicians, appeared oblivious to this practical reality: a patient, subjected to several months of unsuccessful dietary treatment, will often defect from medical follow-up. Such an outcome denies the physician the opportunity to prescribe effective treatment with a drug.

In the 1993 NCEP guidelines, the Expert Panel softened its stance on diet. No longer did the Panel insist on dietary treatment for six months. Instead, the report agreed to starting a drug "after an *adequate trial* of dietary therapy." Nevertheless, the Panel still labels diet and exercise "safer and less expensive." [Never mind that they are not effective in reaching the goals of treatment!]

What Can Be Accomplished
If Doctors Are Good At Niacin?

Why don't more doctors use niacin, preferring instead lovastatin or its related compounds? Mainly because many doctors are *not good at niacin*, and they believe the assertions of *niacin detractors* (who include not only the diet advocates but also the sales representatives of companies selling competing drugs) that niacin is difficult to manage or has serious toxic effects. This book will teach you why those assertions are incorrect.

With more widespread use of niacin, countless lives would be saved by preventing heart attacks and strokes. These serious cardiovascular events then would not disturb or destroy the quality of life for so many people. The need for expensive and dangerous cardiac surgery and other invasive methods of treatment would be lessened, expensive hospitalization reduced, and tremendous expenditures on other cholesterol-control drugs avoided. Remember that heart attacks are preventable. From now on, a heart attack should be regarded as a therapeutic failure. So should strokes and other artery-blocking catastrophes.

All this could be accomplished at modest expense and without the *toxic effects and side effects of diet*. Diet advocates are fond of saying that "all drugs have side effects and toxic effects," implying that diet does not. Diet actually has both side effects and toxic effects, if you stop to think about it.

Diet's *toxic effects* are the heart attacks and strokes which occur when diet fails to control cholesterol adequately. The *side effects* are the worry, concern, and guilt which the public, brainwashed by the diet advocates and the media, experiences when buying food, eating food, cooking food, or even thinking about food.

How can we make the vast majority of physicians *good at niacin?* You are reading the book which makes this possible.

Summary

◆ To lessen the exorbitant toll in deaths and reduced quality of life from atherosclerotic cardiovascular disease, mainly heart attacks and strokes, patients and their physicians must be aware of coronary risk factors. Abnormal factors should be treated to reduce risk, either primary prevention (before a serious event) or secondary prevention (after an event).

◆ The day has arrived when a heart attack should be considered a therapeutic failure.

◆ Diet is a weak and often ineffective method of cholesterol control.

◆ Niacin's advantages are not matched by any other agents. No drug or other measure favorably affects any of several recently discovered benefits of niacin.

◆ Niacin's clinical benefits include reducing heart attacks, strokes and related events, cardiovascular surgery, cardiovascular hospitalization, and all hospitalization.

◆ Niacin's benefits in serum lipids include reducing total and bad (LDL) cholesterol, increasing good (HDL) cholesterol, reducing triglycerides, reducing Lp(a), increasing the ratio of HDL_2 to HDL_3, and converting small-particle LDLC to large-particle LDLC. All these changes tend to reduce arterial deposits which lead to heart attacks, strokes, and other atherosclerotic complications.

◆ Niacin is the only inexpensive drug for cholesterol control, roughly one-sixth to one-tenth the cost of other current agents.

◆ The public and medical profession have not heard more about niacin's value because it is not patentable. No single company can reap large profits from its exclusive sale.

◆ The manufacturers of the expensive drugs are competing in multi-million dollar advertising campaigns aimed at the public as well as the medical profession, seeking larger shares of the multi-billion dollar market. They are not likely to reduce the prices of their products soon.

◆ If all doctors were good at niacin, more than 90% of persons who need cholesterol control could be taking niacin rather than the expensive drugs. This would reduce by billions of dollars each year the expenditures on drugs for cholesterol control.

◆ Patients and their doctors should take part in a gradual revolution, leading to more widespread use of niacin rather than the expensive agents, while prevailing on the medical profession and HMO's to recognize its advantages and favor its use.

CHAPTER THREE

Assessing Risk Factors and Applying Guidelines

Now let's get down to the important questions of whether you, or some one close to you, might be in the 29% of American adults who should receive treatment for abnormal cholesterol fractions. Your physician must be involved from the start, not only to order the needed laboratory tests but also to take your blood pressure to see whether this other important risk factor requires treatment. The tests needed are the total cholesterol (TC), plus good and bad cholesterol fractions (LDLC and HDLC), which make up the "lipid profile."

What Blood Pressure Levels Need To Be Treated?

High blood pressure *never produces any symptoms.* However, it does lead to strokes and heart attacks, the symptoms of which could be your first clue that blood pressure is excessive unless you have regular check-ups and follow your doctor's advice to control hypertension. Blood pressure should be controlled to less than 140 for the systolic (upper number of the blood pressure) and less than 90 for the diastolic (lower number). We once thought that the natural increase in the upper number with aging ("100 plus your age") was acceptable, but further study has shown that lowering this value to a target level below 140 reduces the number of heart attacks and strokes, especially strokes.

There are numerous excellent drugs available to treat high blood pressure. Unfortunately, many physicians tend to choose one of the newer, expensive drugs as first-line treatment. The wise policy of the Joint National Council on Hypertension is to start treatment with one of two types of drugs, either a diuretic or a beta-blocker. Both of these are time-proven winners, available generically and inexpensively. Beta-blockers are an especially good choice in persons with a previous heart attack or with significant risk factors. Several studies more than two decades ago showed that beta-blockers reduce the risk of heart attack.

Once you know your blood pressure and your bad and good cholesterol fractions, you and your doctor are in a position to assess your coronary risk factors, which estimate your chances of developing coronary disease or related atherosclerotic conditions.

Your Risk Factor Score

Score one risk factor for each of the following situations:

- Male or postmenopausal female
- Family history of heart attack or stroke in a close male relative before age 50 or close female relative before age 60
- Current smoker
- High blood pressure
- LDL (bad) cholesterol is too high or HDL (good) cholesterol is too low
- Diabetic
- Physically inactive (failure to walk 30 minutes three or more times a week)
- Obese (more than 30% above ideal weight)

Reduce your risk factor score by one if:

- HDL (good) cholesterol above 60

Who Needs Treatment for Cholesterol Problems?

Now that you and your doctor have listed your risk factors, or you have done the same for some one close to you, how do you know whose cholesterol levels need to be treated? This requires knowing bad and good cholesterol fractions (LDLC and HDLC) and application of the NCEP guidelines. In some instances we use the "Parsons Simplified Guidelines" (PSG) when the NCEP "Expert Panel" has not been specific.

At What Level Does Bad (LDL) Cholesterol Need To Be Treated?

First, have you had a heart attack or other event which tells us you definitely have artery narrowing or blockage? The list includes:

Rob   *SANDY*

No • Heart attack (myocardial infarction)   *NO*

No • Angina pectoris (pain from heart muscle)   *NO*

No • Coronary artery bypass   *NO*

No • Other interventional procedure to open obstructed heart arteries, such   *NO*
as balloon angioplasty, stent (device to hold artery open),
atherectomy (removing obstructing plaque from an artery by a rotary
cutting device), or thrombolytic therapy (dripping a "clot-busting"
drug into the blocked artery as a clot is developing)

No • Leg pain due to reduced circulation   *No*

No • Surgery on neck or leg arteries   *No*

If the answer is "yes" to any of these situations, a special guideline applies to you. The *LDL cholesterol* should be reduced to *less than 100*. The 1993 NCEP guidelines added this recommendation because such levels not only reduce new cholesterol deposits but also lead to regression of some existing plaques.

If you have none of the above situations, the LDLC target is not so demanding. NCEP advises *LDLC less than 130* for persons with two or more risk factors but accepts *less than 160* for those with fewer than two risk factors. I consider it my job to simplify life for my patients, not make it more complicated. The Parsons Simplified Guidelines (PSG) like to see *LDLC less than 130 for everyone.*

At What Level Does Good (HDL) Cholesterol Need To Be Treated?

The 1993 NCEP guidelines correctly state that HDLC levels below 35 are dangerous because they increase the risk of heart attack (and presumably all other events due to arterial narrowing). However, they fail to specify a target level. Obviously, just getting the HDLC level to 36 would not be good enough. How much of a cushion above 35 should we seek? The PSG recommend HDLC of *45 or higher*. Sometimes we have to settle for above 40.

39

At this point you know, with your doctor's help, whether you need treatment for cholesterol problems. If you have not had an atherosclerotic event (the above list) and have a satisfactory lipid profile, enjoy life and resolve to recheck the lipid profile in three years. If you are among the 29% of American adults whose cholesterol patterns need treatment by the current guidelines we just reviewed, see your doctor. But first you should read the following chapters to learn why diet is usually not effective and why physicians should use niacin, which is by far the best treatment for most lipid problems. You will learn how I would treat you if you were my patient. This knowledge will enable you to recognize whether your physician is good at niacin and help him to acquire this skill if he has not already developed it. It can assure the best of all situations for successful treatment: a knowledgeable doctor and an informed patient.

CHAPTER FOUR

Why Not Diet to
Control Cholesterol?

Why not use diet to treat everyone with abnormal cholesterol fractions?
It all boils down to three simple facts:

1. Diet is usually ineffective in reaching the stated goals.

2. If diet lowers total and LDL cholesterol at all, it usually does so
    only during periods of weight reduction.

3. Diet is unnecessary. Niacin accomplishes the goals better in the
    presence of an ordinary American diet.

Why doesn't diet usually work? Why is it a waste of time, frustrating to
both patient and physician? Expressed in simple, homespun terms, the serum
cholesterol depends on what the *body factory* is doing, not what one eats.
(Serum is the liquid part of blood, when all the blood cells are removed. It is
more correct to speak of *serum* cholesterol rather than *blood* cholesterol, so
that's what we will do from now on.)

Think in these terms: the body manufactures about 80% of the
cholesterol in serum and body tissues, with only about 20% coming from
food. Everyone inherits a different body factory. Although you may eat
identical diets, your neighbor can have a perfect cholesterol pattern while you
have much too much bad (LDL) cholesterol. Because LDLC is the largest
fraction, LDLC and total cholesterol (TC) vary together. When LDLC is high,
TC is also high. We don't need to consider HDLC when talking about diet,
because *diet has no effect on HDLC*. A person whose body factory is not
making enough HDLC cannot be helped by diet.

A distinguished cholesterol researcher, Dr. Gordon Gould, was

41

chairman of the AHA's Council on Arteriosclerosis in the late 1950's. His presidential address to the elite of cholesterol research contained an insightful comment on the role of the body factory, as he observed, "It's as though we went into a house and found that it was too hot. So far we are trying to decide what we should throw into the furnace when we should be looking for the thermostat."

George Mann, now retired, had an outstanding career in cholesterol research at Vanderbilt University. In his book, mentioned earlier, he contends that diet is not effective in cholesterol reduction except during periods of weight reduction—"and you can't go on losing weight forever." I have never taken the position that diet always fails to control cholesterol, but I do say that *diet is a weak and often ineffective method.*

In my opinion the NCEP guidelines of 1988 were wrong when they specified six months of diet before considering medication. The Panel recommended starting with the AHA Step One diet; then, if cholesterol levels had not been controlled after three months, they advised *making the diet stricter.* There are only two reasons for failure of the Step One diet after three months. Perhaps the patient has not been following the diet, finding it onerous and certainly not acceptable for the rest of his life. In that case, making the diet stricter will also be doomed to failure. Or the patient's metabolic defect (in the body factory) is too great to be controlled by the Step One diet. If so, there is a good possibility that the next step, a stricter diet, will also fail—or may be unacceptable to the patient, even if he endured the Step One program.

Remember the Diet-Heart Feasibility Trial of the early 1960's? It showed that people would not follow any diet with significant limitation of fat and cholesterol; furthermore, it did not make much difference if they did. If that elaborate study, with everything going for it, failed to demonstrate that diet was an effective and practical method for cholesterol control, what study could? No wonder the diet advocates have swept its results under the rug!

Coronary Heart Disease:
The Dietary Sense and Nonsense

This was the title of a symposium held in Washington, D.C. a few years ago and then the title of the book based on the symposium. I have already mentioned the book and its editor, George Mann, who organized the symposium. The book is still available for any readers desiring more scientific detail regarding the futility of diet. It is understandable to the lay reader and, of course, to doctors and dietitians as well. The book consists of eight chapters, each a forty-minute talk at the meeting, with lively discussions after every two papers. There were seven speakers. When one of the invited participants canceled because of surgery a few weeks before the meeting, George filled the gap with a talk on her assigned topic.

The speakers and several like-minded members of the audience, who contributed their thinking in the discussion periods, call themselves the *Veritas Society*, from the Latin word for *truth*. They felt strongly that the American people (including the medical profession) had long been brainwashed by advocates of the Diet-Heart theory and should be taught the real facts.

The Veritas Society's symposium was conceived as a media event. When the idea was first hatched at a meeting in Sweden a year earlier, Mann and others agreed that dissemination of misleading information by diet advocates was a worldwide phenomenon. Speakers who were Irish, Czech, and a New Zealander represented this international aspect. I was not one of the original planners but was privileged to join the group a few months before the meeting and give the final talk of the day, *Clinical Alternatives*. In essence, after a day in which other speakers revealed the shortcomings and false allegations about diet, I addressed the question, "If not diet, then what?" The answer was, of course, cholesterol control by appropriate drugs, especially niacin.

All Veritas participants were scientists who have devoted their careers to atherosclerosis research. The discussions between their papers are spirited and candid, naming names and citing organizations involved in the concerted effort to perpetuate the emphasis on diet. This is not a conspiracy, really, in the sense that dietary advocates and the food industry ever sat down and hatched a plan to brainwash the public, but that has been the effect.

The symposium had been widely announced to the news media. Representatives of leading news organizations and magazines had assured George Mann (and me, in one instance—*People* magazine) that they would have reporters there. However, media coverage at the symposium was meager at best. Where was the media? The reason for their absence was discovered within days after the meeting but edited into the book as a question and answer in the final discussion. Two days before the meeting some one had placed a false report on the East Coast news wires that the symposium had been canceled! Clearly, this "dirty trick" was the work of an organization sufficiently worried about the effect of the message that they felt it necessary to go to this extreme. In the book, replying to "Who did that?" George says,

"We are not sure, but it must be obvious that what we are doing here today is perceived by segments of the food and drug industries to be threatening."

Actually, there had been earlier indications that the Veritas symposium was considered threatening by organizations relating to foods, drugs, and research in general. A British scientist, scheduled as a speaker, had to cancel when his employer, the Medical Research Council (roughly the equivalent of our FDA) forbade him to participate. A well-known cardiologist-researcher in the U.S. also withdrew as a speaker when NHLBI (National Heart, Lung, and Blood Institute), a branch of NIH, informed him that a proposal he had submitted would be in serious jeopardy if he took part in the symposium.

Telling me about these events as he was pulling the program together, George Mann announced, regarding his anonymous opponents, "They are really playing hardball!" Thus the newswire "dirty trick" came as no surprise. Nevertheless, it was disillusioning that scientists, speaking the truth, could not present their information to the media and, through the media, to the public— all because of the dishonesty of the unknown opposition. One wonders what their reaction to this book will be.

You Don't Have To Diet To Control Cholesterol!

Besides the fact that diet is weak and often ineffective in treatment of cholesterol abnormalities, there is another reason not to use it. *Diet isn't* *necessary!*

In my first study at Mayo Clinic, we used niacin without any change in diet. A few patients had been on fat-restricted diets without any benefit, but results with niacin were equally impressive with and without diet. In my first published Madison report (1957), the summary included, "Prompt and sustained reduction of blood cholesterol levels was obtained in nearly all of the hypercholesteremic patients who received large doses of nicotinic acid...No dietary restrictions were imposed in this study." Again (1959), this time from Madison: "All patients were instructed to continue to eat as they had eaten before the study. Except for one man on a low-fat diet and three patients on diabetic diets, all patients were eating typical American diets." In my papers and those from the Mayo Clinic, this fact was repeated over and over. *Niacin produces its significant changes in serum cholesterol in the presence of an ordinary American diet.* Although my slogan was not coined until 1991, it was already apparent in the late fifties that *You don't have to diet to control cholesterol!*

Eggs: To Eat or Not To Eat

Until recently the customary dietary advice for cholesterol problems, reduced to its simplest terms, has been: "Cut down on fats and don't eat eggs." Let's talk about eggs.

Egg yolks represent the greatest source of cholesterol in the diet (not fat, just cholesterol). When it first became apparent (late 1940's, early 1950's?) that serum cholesterol was related to the development of atherosclerosis, a natural thought was that limiting cholesterol-containing foods (mainly eggs) should reduce serum levels. It didn't work. For many years I sat in the annual meetings of cholesterol researchers who would report their studies in animals, trying to decide whether cholesterol in the diet was important or not. The results were conflicting. One study would say that adding cholesterol increased serum levels; another would say that it did not. I was impressed that, after so many studies over so many years, investigators still couldn't be sure whether dietary cholesterol made any difference. To me, this made it clear: *Dietary cholesterol doesn't make any difference!* (I also asked myself why they were spending their time doing animal experiments when the animals we were really interested in—humans—were readily available for study.)

When a new patient entered my Madison studies, I would pointedly say to continue eating exactly as before the study. We did not suggest becoming fat; if already fat, losing would be nice, but I made no specific recommendations. We wanted to know the effect of niacin, not niacin plus some sort of dietary intervention. As expected, no one lost weight significantly.

The response of many patients to this no-diet approach was, "Do you mean I may eat eggs?" My uniform reaction was, "You haven't been eating eggs?" A typical reply: "I haven't eaten an egg in four years." Nowadays there's another variation: "I use only [name of a popular egg substitute]." This allowed me to muse, "Let's see: you haven't eaten an egg in four years and your doctor has referred you to my study because your cholesterol level is 315. Has avoiding eggs achieved your goal or not?"

Another approach to the egg question in a skeptical patient is the "egg test." If a person has been eating no eggs, we do a baseline blood test, including LDLC and HDLC fractions; then I encourage eating eggs liberally for a month. Two or three a day is not out of the question. After a month, we recheck the lipid profile. I have never seen the cholesterol level change significantly in the relatively few times I have done this. Why only a few times? Because most people tend to accept my simple explanation and are pleased to hear that a medication will make it unnecessary to diet, so they don't want to waste time proving further that eating eggs does not change cholesterol.

In 1992 Vorster and associates in South Africa reported a persuasive study which was really a carefully done egg test. They examined the effect of egg intake on cholesterol and the lipoprotein profile in 70 healthy men, ages 18 and 19, who were randomly assigned to eat either three, seven, or fourteen eggs a week for five months. At the end of the study, there were *no significant differences in serum lipids and lipoproteins* among the three groups. The authors concluded, therefore, that limitation of eggs in the diet is not necessary or worthwhile. I advise my patients to eat all the eggs they desire since eggs are an excellent source of protein and do not change the cholesterol picture. There is absolutely no justification for buying any of the expensive products made from egg whites only or for discarding yolks, as some persons do.

Some diet advocates would say that a small percentage of adults are "egg-sensitive," meaning that eggs raise their cholesterol levels significantly for some unknown reason, obviously having to do with the body factory. An egg test would identify such persons, but this really doesn't matter since niacin controls total and LDL cholesterol in these few patients as well as in others, who comprise the vast majority. There have been other studies in recent years that also show very little change, if any, when eggs are added to the diet under controlled conditions.

The leader of a 1995 AHA conference on diet and cholesterol, Robert Nicolosi (Lowell, Massachusetts) summarized, "For the majority of people, taking eggs out of the diet does nothing." That's what I meant when I started this section by saying, "*Until recently*, the customary dietary advice has been..." There has been a gradual drift away from the old guard AHA advice, but without fanfare. George Mann is right; no one likes to admit he has been wrong all those years.

Is High-Fiber Diet an Effective Way to Reduce Cholesterol Levels?

Diet high in fiber can lower total and LDL cholesterol a little bit but not really enough to make any difference if one has levels in the range which need treatment. Such a program has no effect on HDLC. Total cholesterol reductions are less than 10%, which will seldom reach the goals of treatment unless the problem is very mild. It is not clear whether fiber acts on its own or just replaces fats and other foods with more calories. Psyllium seed, the bulk-forming preparation to alter bowel function (Metamucil, numerous other brand names) also can reduce cholesterol a little, but the same comments apply. Soluble fiber, as in oat bran, may be a little better. All in all, it is not worth considering high fiber diet as an important part of treatment if one needs significant cholesterol reduction. Use fiber to improve bowel function; treat hypercholesteremia with a drug which really reaches the goals.

Trans-Fatty Acids: Butter or Margarine?

Another issue being debated in recent years is whether *trans*-fatty acids (TFA) play a significant role in development of atherosclerosis. TFA are altered fats produced when liquid vegetable oils are solidified in production of margarine, making them more spreadable. George Mann, while decrying the usual dietary advice about fat and cholesterol, is a leading protester against TFA. He speculates that the increase in coronary disease in the twentieth century parallels the increased use of margarines.

In the last several decades there certainly has been a huge promotional effort to convert American eating from saturated fatty acids (as in animal fats) to unsaturated fatty acids (in vegetable oils). Many dietary advocates have recommended margarines, whose oils are originally unsaturated when in the liquid state, in preference to butter, with its saturated fatty acids of animal origin. There are two flaws in this type of advice. One is that replacing saturated fatty acids with polyunsaturated fatty acids became outmoded when this proved to be ineffective at reducing cholesterol. The other is that converting liquid vegetable oils to more solid margarines requires that most of the unsaturated fatty acids be saturated, so one does not get much unsaturated fat from margarine.

Whether this TFA production is harmful has not been resolved. As a clinician my job is to simplify life for my patients, not complicate it. If the TFA question comes up, I tell them that the final word isn't in. Since butter tastes better, why not go ahead and eat butter? Of course, if weight reduction is a goal, one should *avoid both butter and margarine* because they are equally high in calories. Omitting all table spreads from the diet is not difficult and eliminates a significant number of calories.

Red Meat: Enjoy It

What about eating red meat? Many persons somehow have gotten the idea that avoiding red meat is helpful in cholesterol control. It is not unusual for a new patient in my office to announce proudly that in their household they eat no red meat or only have it occasionally. This automatically wins them a copy of an attractive brochure titled *Mealstyles*, which explains that eating lean red meat is all right. The booklet includes a series of beautifully illustrated international recipes. I turn the brochure over and show its back cover to the patient. The American Beef Council co-sponsors it. No surprise. But look at this other sponsor, whose name appears above that of the Beef Council: the American Heart Association![1]

The message of *Mealstyles* is simple. *Lean* red meat poses no health problem of any sort. If there is any caution, it should be to avoid the fat in or around the meat. On its last page, the booklet lists "Beef's Skinniest Six," those cuts which contain the least fat. These are the nicest cuts, which you would buy anyhow. The booklet advises trimming all the fat you can and then broiling, in most instances. In fact, studies have shown that lean beef and chicken have the same effects on TC, LDLC, HDLC, and triglycerides. These two types of meat are interchangeable in the AHA Step One Diet. So eating red meat is perfectly acceptable. *Enjoy it.*

Vegetarian Diets: Not Advised To Reduce Atherosclerosis

What about vegetarian diets? Vegetarians adopt this preference for various reasons. If the reason has anything to do with prevention of atherosclerotic disease, some facts from a chapter by Mary Enig, Ph.D. (Silver Spring, Maryland) in George Mann's book may lead vegetarians to reconsider.

After noting that vegetarians are said to have significantly lower cholesterol levels than others, Dr. Enig calls attention to several little-known facts. Both male and female vegetarians have *lower HDL (good) cholesterol*, an undesirable situation. Male vegetarians have *lower* mortality from coronary heart disease than male non-vegetarians, but they have *equal* death rates from all causes. Female vegetarians, on the other hand, have *higher*

---

[1] Do not be surprised that I use this endorsement to illustrate the value of *Mealstyles* and of eating red meat, even though I have criticized AHA for its strong advocacy of dietary treatment of hypercholesteremia over the years. AHA is a worthwhile organization that has done more than any other to further the care of cardiovascular diseases. If it were not for the good-old-boy group of diet advocates and their unbending insistence that diet effectively controls cholesterol, I would be an unqualified AHA booster.

coronary mortality than female nonvegetarians and *much higher* all-cause mortality. Furthermore, autopsy studies have shown that vegetarians have *just as much atherosclerosis* as nonvegetarians, even though the vegetarians have lower serum cholesterol levels. Conclusion: if the goal is prevention of heart attack and other atherosclerotic disease, a vegetarian diet is not the answer.

Dean Ornish (San Francisco) has been an advocate of a strict vegetarian diet as part of a complicated program to reduce heart disease. With numerous associates he conducted "The Lifestyle Heart Trial," which assigned 28 patients to an experimental group and 20 to a usual-care group, then followed them for a year. The former group was asked to follow a very low-fat vegetarian diet, plus several other interventions to reduce stress and provide exercise. Before starting the study, patients had recently had coronary angiograms and were willing to have this procedure repeated a year later.

The diet provided fruits, vegetables, grains, legumes, and soy bean products without caloric restriction. No animal products were allowed except one egg white and one cup of non-fat milk or yogurt each day. Stress management techniques included stretching exercises, breathing techniques, meditation, progressive relaxation, and imagery. Patients were asked to practice these techniques for at least one hour a day. Exercise, usually walking, was prescribed according to baseline treadmill performance, advising a minimum of three hours a week in sessions of at least thirty minutes.

Twice-weekly group discussions provided social support to help patients adhere to the lifestyle change program. These were led by a clinical psychologist, who "facilitated discussions of strategies for maintaining adherence to the program, communication skills, and expression of feelings about relationships at work and at home." Adherence to the various components of the lifestyle program was said to be excellent. During the year of the trial, the experimental group had reductions in TC (24%) and LDLC (37%). HDLC did not change in either group.

Analysis of coronary arteriograms before the trial and after one year showed a little reduction of lesions in the experimental group and a little average progression in the control group. Five men in the control group also showed slight regression of atherosclerosis. They were said to have exercised more often and for longer periods, plus consuming fewer calories and less cholesterol than the control patients who showed progression of atherosclerosis.

Ornish and his colleagues correctly questioned whether such comprehensive lifestyle changes could be sustained in larger populations of patients with coronary disease. They state, "The point of our study was to determine what is true, not what is practicable." They further observe that "adherence to this lifestyle program needs to be very good for overall regression to occur."

My reaction as a practicing physician is that this bizarre program will appeal only to a very small segment of the population. The key word is "lifestyle." Who wants a week full of such time-consuming interventions that it leaves little time for really living?

Ornish has shown that reduction in coronary artery lesions can occur in a small group willing to suffer a strange and demanding program, but does not know the relative contribution of each component. As in all regression studies, the changes in diameters of arteries were small, which makes their significance questionable. Patients I know will almost unanimously choose a program that allows a normal American diet and requires just a few pills each day, under knowledgeable medical supervision.

Comparison of Diet with Niacin

Among my studies in Madison around 1960 was a simple comparison of diet with a modest dose (500 mg three times a day) of an intermediate-release niacin product, aluminum nicotinate (Nicalex, Walker Laboratories). The active ingredient, niacin, was loosely attached to aluminum hydroxide, the same compound widely used as an antacid, except that in this situation it did not have that effect. This loose binding delayed niacin's absorption perhaps 90 minutes, enough to prevent flushing.

After preparing them with a sufficient placebo interval to produce a baseline average, we divided 60 patients into four groups of 15. Table 7 shows the plan of study and results. One group was instructed in diet (the equivalent of the AHA Step One diet) and used it throughout the 24-week study, with no medication. A second group also used diet throughout, but for the second 12 weeks we added Nicalex. The third group started with Nicalex and no diet; then diet was added for the second 12 weeks. The fourth group used both diet and Nicalex throughout both 12-week periods.

We can summarize the results by saying that *the major falls in cholesterol occurred when the niacin product was used.* The group on diet alone had almost no reduction in cholesterol (326 to 318 in 12 weeks, with no further fall in the second period). Group 2 also showed minimal reduction

(332 to 328, not significant) in the first period but the average cholesterol level fell from 328 to 290 (-38) when niacin was added. Group 3 showed a large reduction on Nicalex alone, 321 to 271 (-50), with a lesser further reduction after adding diet (271 to 256). Group 4 showed prompt reduction on the combined program of diet and Nicalex, 328 to 280 (-48), which remained stable (276) on the same treatment in the second period.

To reiterate, the major reductions occurred when niacin was used; practically nothing happened on diet alone. This study was a formal demonstration of what I had already decided from clinical observations. The large body of evidence in the Veritas symposium gave more scientific backing to my summary statement: *Diet is a weak and often ineffective method for cholesterol control.*

Table 7
Effect of Diet and Aluminum Nicotinate on Serum Cholesterol

	Before	First Period		Second Period	
Group 1	326	Diet	318	Diet	318
Group 2	332	Diet	328	Diet + AlN	290
Group 3	321	AlN	271	AlN + Diet	256
Group 4	328	Diet + AlN	280	Diet + AlN	276

Study of diet and/or aluminum nicotinate (AlN), (Nicalex, Walker Laboratories) in four groups of 15 patients each, treated for two 12-week periods. See text for details.

What Do I Recommend About Diet?

If a person in need of cholesterol control also needs to lose weight, restriction of calories is the only way to reach this goal. As a rule it is best to proceed with a niacin program for cholesterol control at the same time. Why? Unless the cholesterol abnormality is very mild, diet will probably not attain the goals of treatment. As mentioned earlier, some improvement may occur during weight reduction, only to disappear during subsequent weight maintenance. Of course, there is also another possibility, that the patient will not succeed in losing weight at all. In any event, it is best to treat the cholesterol problem separately, on its own merits.

51

Suppose a person simply wants to try diet first, hoping to avoid the need for medications. I have no problem with this, but the patient should know three things:

- Two months is long enough to determine whether diet will control the cholesterol problem or approach the goals.

- The diet she follows for those two months must be a program she is willing to follow from now on.

- It is not necessary to diet to control cholesterol.

Of course, diet applies only if the cholesterol problem is *too much bad cholesterol*, which results in *too high total cholesterol*. If the problem is *not enough good cholesterol*, diet is not helpful.

Some persons with mixed hyperlipidemia, a combination of elevated serum cholesterol and triglycerides, may respond to diet, especially if combined with obesity, as it often is. However, one should know that niacin is the NCEP-recommended drug of choice for mixed hyperlipidemia. It should be the drug of choice for every lipid problem.

Summary

◆ Diet is usually a weak and ineffective approach for control of LDLC or HDLC levels. If diet helps at all, it reduces only the LDLC level and usually only during periods of weight reduction.

◆ For cholesterol control, diet is unnecessary. Niacin reduces LDLC and increases HDLC levels in the presence of an ordinary American diet.

◆ Diet has little to do with serum cholesterol levels. Intake of cholesterol, mainly in eggs, has nothing to do with the serum cholesterol and lipoprotein cholesterol levels.

◆ An important feasibility study showed that even highly motivated participants would not follow diets with any significant amount of fat restriction; furthermore, it did not make much difference if they did.

◆ Dietary advocates (researchers in this field, the American Heart Association, National Institutes of Health, and especially the food industry) have brainwashed the media over the years.

◆ The media in turn has brainwashed the American public, including the medical profession.

◆ Eating butter is all right unless you prefer the flavor or cost of margarine.

◆ Eating lean red meat does not adversely affect serum cholesterol levels.

◆ Vegetarian eating may result in lower cholesterol levels but has adverse effects on HDLC. Vegetarians of both sexes have all-cause mortality equal to or greater than nonvegetarians. In autopsy studies, vegetarians have as much atherosclerosis as nonvegetarians.

◆ The bizarre program used by Ornish and associates in their "lifestyle" trial, although interesting to read about, has no practical value.

CHAPTER FIVE

The Important Differences Between Plain and Time-Release Niacin

Teaching patients and their doctors what I know about niacin must begin with the important differences between *plain* and *time-release* niacin. The FDA distinction between these classes of products depends on how long it takes a tablet to dissolve in a standard test. To perform this test they suspend tablets in a wire basket in a container of swirling water at a standard temperature. If the tablets dissolve in less than one hour, the product is called *plain* (or sometimes *compressed tablets,* but we will use the simpler term). If a tablet takes longer than an hour to dissolve, it is called *time-release.*

Plain Niacin

When we first worked with niacin in 1955 and the next few years, the only available product was plain niacin. When one takes plain niacin (NA) by mouth, whether in doses as small as 50 mg or as large as 3000 mg, the drug dissolves rapidly and is absorbed almost immediately. In the FDA test, the tablets dissolve in only three to five minutes. Even doses less than 50 mg can cause prompt cutaneous (skin) flushing, due to marked dilatation (widening) of the capillaries, the tiny blood vessels in the skin. Larger doses, even 1000 mg or more, *do not* cause a more severe flush than 50 to 100 mg. The flush may be confined to the head and neck; it can involve the upper half of the body, or occasionally the whole body surface. The skin turns red when its capillaries dilate. The person feels hot in the affected area, which may also tingle or itch. Sometimes small bumps, like mini-hives, appear on the trunk or arms, going away when the flush subsides. The flush lasts perhaps 15 to 20 minutes, occasionally as long as 45 to 60 minutes, or (very rarely) even longer.

Although this may sound terrible, it really isn't. Here's why. When the dose of plain niacin is 1000 mg three times a day (the starting dose the Canadians used, as we did in our early studies), the flush is most severe on the first day, especially with the first dose. Remember, the flush is no more severe with 1000 mg than with 50 mg. As the drug is continued in full dosage, the flush diminishes with each day and even with each dose. Before long *the flush will, for all practical purposes, disappear.* The average time is *three to four days,* as reported by the Canadian originators of the idea and confirmed in my Rochester and Madison studies of the late 1950's.

The flush is only a nuisance; it is not serious. It does not affect heart rate and blood pressure. The flush does not aggravate or cause chest pain of coronary disease (called *angina pectoris* or simply *angina).* Each patient should be fully informed, by oral and printed discussions, of the natural history of the flush, emphasizing that it almost always subsides early in treatment.

Despite this, some patients will be distressed enough to call the physician. A doctor good at niacin will calmly and confidently remind the patient of the importance of continuing full dosage until the flush is no longer troublesome. This is what I did in 1955, armed with Dr. Hoffer's assurance that the flush disappeared early. Likewise, present-day doctors can do the same, based on more than forty years of further experience since then.

My observations in the early years taught me facts about the flush which hold true today:

- When telling how the flush subsides, I usually add "for practical purposes" because some persons will still feel a flicker at times.

- The first dose of the day may sometimes cause a little flushing, milder and briefer than at first.

- The same may occur after a dose taken with only a small meal.

- Taking plain niacin on an empty stomach can cause more of a flush, so we always advise taking this form in the middle of a meal.

- If one resumes NA after stopping it for a while, flushing may recur but is usually milder than at first.

- *Increasing the size of individual doses does not result in resumption of the flush.* This is fortunate because my early studies showed that about 50% of patients require more than the starting dose of 3000 mg a day to control the cholesterol problem.

Current medical literature commonly advises starting with smaller doses of plain niacin and gradually increasing to the target dose. *This is the best way I know to prolong the flush.* It will almost certainly extend the number of days it takes to subside entirely. For this reason, NA should be taken persistently in the starting dose I have always recommended, 1000 mg three times a day. When authors in recent years have advised starting with a smaller dose and increasing over many weeks, they show lack of basic knowledge of niacin's behavior. Because at least half of patients on NA will need more than 3000 mg per day, in divided dosage, there is no point in using smaller doses initially. Among my observations of the late 1950's was the fact that *a total daily dose of plain niacin as small as 1500 mg is seldom effective.*

Taking an ordinary aspirin tablet (325 mg) each morning will lessen flushing considerably by inhibiting the body's release of prostaglandins, substances which are responsible for the flush. Some have advised taking an aspirin tablet before each dose of niacin, but for most persons a single morning dose suffices, especially if the supervising physician starts with full niacin doses to be sure the flush subsides early. Other prostaglandin inhibitors, such as ibuprofen and related drugs, should also prevent the flush but are more likely to cause stomach problems, including ulcer, possibly with bleeding. The single aspirin tablet should be taken on first arising in the morning with a generous amount of water (six to eight ounces). This dissolves and dilutes the tablet, washing it out of the stomach and encouraging earlier absorption, instead of leaving the tablet on the stomach wall to cause irritation. Aspirin can also irritate the stomach and even cause ulcer, but taking it with this generous amount of water should prevent such a mishap.

Until the flush subsides, especially if the patient has trouble tolerating it, avoiding hot beverages with meals may be advisable. Hot soups, as well as coffee or tea, can increase flushing since they dilate skin capillaries, even without niacin. Alcohol, although it also dilates skin capillaries, has not been a problem in this regard.

In general, flushing tends to be worse in persons who blush easily and in those with red hair or very fair complexions. However, they usually get over the flush as promptly as others. Rarely, a person will go on flushing as long as she uses plain niacin. This can prevent long-term use of the drug, but in more than forty years I have encountered only one or two such patients.

Fortunately, there is an alternative that offers most patients the benefits of niacin without significant flushing.

Time-Release Niacin

Using time-release[1] niacin (TRNA) reduces the severity of the flush and may eliminate it entirely, especially if one takes the morning aspirin. In the late 1950's, several drug companies produced time-release niacin tablets for investigational use (at Mayo Clinic and in Madison). They sought to eliminate the flush, making niacin more acceptable to patients and giving the company a patentable product. These older TRNA products met with varying degrees of success in lessening the flush but tended to cause more nausea and more alteration in liver function tests than plain niacin. None of those preparations is on the market today, but newer and better products are available.

Today there are two types of time-release medications. One is the *beadlets-in-a-capsule* type, originally developed by Smith, Kline and French, who called their products "Spansules."

Some may recall TV commercials for the antihistamine drug Contac, in which beadlets from halves of a capsule fell and bounced in slow motion. In these pellets, active ingredients such as niacin, are coated with materials which dissolve at various rates in the intestine, releasing the drug for intermittent absorption.

I do not recommend the beadlet type of time-release niacin. From the famous Contac ad, one would get the impression that these tiny spheres go through the intestinal tract individually, each dissolving at its own rate, providing delayed and sustained absorption. However, studies from the early 1980's indicated that beadlets move through the intestine as a bolus (clump). Because the pellets did not go their separate ways, the absorption patterns were not as smooth as expected. This may be the reason that beadlet preparations tend to cause more nausea than other TRNA dosage forms.

The other method of delaying absorption is the *wax-matrix* type of tablet first developed by CIBA-Geigy in Slow-K, its time-release potassium tablet. The tablet can best be visualized as a sponge made of wax, with the openings of the sponge filled with the soluble material (potassium chloride in the CIBA product, niacin in several time-release caplets available today). As

---

[1] Tablets or capsules which are absorbed slowly rather than immediately are variously called time-release, sustained-release, delayed-release, gradual release, continuous-release, or prolonged-release. These terms are not exactly synonymous; there are technical differences, used mainly in the pharmaceutical industry. Because these small distinctions don't matter to the reader or to me, in this book any product which takes more than an hour to dissolve and be absorbed will be called *time-release*, as in time-release niacin, which I abbreviate *TRNA*. This abbreviation is an old one that goes back to my early years of work with the drug.

the caplet passes through the intestine, the very soluble niacin leaches out of the openings of the sponge-like shell and is thus gradually absorbed. Occasionally the wax shell appears in the stool, leading patients to think they have not received the benefit of niacin. The physician should tell patients about this possibility and assure them that the active ingredient has been absorbed.

Some patients feel no flush at all from TRNA, especially if they take a 325 mg aspirin tablet on arising each morning. Some feel mild warmth or tingling at one time or another, but this is usually infrequent and seldom troublesome. When one swallows *plain* niacin, a strong flush occurs almost immediately because the product dissolves so rapidly (three to five minutes in the standard FDA test). With TRNA, which takes hours for its niacin contents to dissolve, any flush is mild and occurs later, often after several hours. One manufacturer tells me that TRNA is better absorbed when taken with food, but I tell patients they may take it at any time, even on an empty stomach if they wish. Patients find this out for themselves as they take TRNA. They also find out that the morning aspirin trick is not needed after a while.

Today's time-release niacin products are approximately twice as potent in their effects on cholesterol and on liver function as plain niacin, presumably because gradual absorption provides more sustained blood levels. This means that niacin works more hours of the day on the liver, the body's main cholesterol factory. By contrast, plain niacin is rapidly absorbed, reaching a higher peak, but then is rapidly removed from the blood. Because of the difference in their potency, if changing from *plain* niacin to a *time-release* product for any reason, it is important that *doses be reduced about in half.* The physician must emphasize this to each patient, cautioning against ill-advised or inadvertent changes in the type of product unless specifically advised and supervised by the doctor.

Thus comparable doses would be 1000 mg three times a day for NA and 500 mg three times a day for TRNA. Failure to understand the dosage relationship of plain vs. time-release niacin can result in serious adverse reactions. Even in equivalent doses, TRNA is somewhat more likely to cause nausea and/or alteration in liver function tests than NA. A subsequent chapter will discuss how to manage side effects.

There are a number of TRNA products on the market today. Because such products have somewhat different absorption patterns and perhaps different clinical characteristics, no physician can possibly be thoroughly familiar with all of them. Switching from one to another without the doctor's knowledge, can lead to trouble with one product which has not occurred with another. For this reason, I advise each doctor to become experienced with one or two TRNA products and *insist that patients use only those.*

In general, my experience and the medical literature regarding TRNA products have shown that each has about the same effect on lipid metabolism. For various reasons I have narrowed my use to one or two. Some are just too high in price. As mentioned above, I do not advise use of any beadlet preparation. Because of reports which may indicate greater side effects, it is probably best to avoid TRNA products purchased in "health food" stores.

My current favorite TRNA is Endur-acin[2], a wax-matrix caplet made by Endurance Products Company of Tigard, Oregon. Until a few years ago I recommended Slo-Niacin, (Upsher-Smith, Minneapolis), which has a patented release mechanism, using a "polygel" matrix rather than wax. The polygel shell is more likely to appear in the stool than that of wax matrix products. One study showed that in seven hours, Endur-acin caplets dissolved more completely, 98% to 99%, compared to 88% for Slo-Niacin and 76% for a beadlet preparation.

Actually, Endur-acin and Slo-Niacin have both performed well for me, but there is a significant difference in their prices. Our recent survey showed that 100 caplets of 500 mg Slo-Niacin cost the patient $13.50, compared to $8.99 for Endur-acin. At an average dose of three to four caplets a day, this brings the monthly cost to $8.09 to $10.78 for Endur-acin vs. $12.15 to $16.20 for Slo-Niacin. If Endur-acin is not available in some pharmacies, the company has a very efficient mail order operation, with attractive pricing.

A New "Plain" Intermediate-Release Product

A recent arrival on the market is a new "plain" niacin tablet made by the manufacturer of Endur-acin. Remember that any tablet which dissolves in less than an hour by the FDA dissolution test is designated as "plain" and anything dissolving in more than an hour called "time-release?" (Sometimes "sustained-release" is used, as on Endur-acin bottles.) By altering the time-release mechanism, Endurance Products managed to reduce the dissolution

---

[2] The registered trademark of Innovite, Inc. of Tigard, Oregon, for this product is ENDUR-ACIN, spelled in all capital letters. After this recognition of that fact, I shall proceed to use the name in my text as "Endur-acin." This decision arises from my intention to mention the drug by name from time to time without making the book look like a commercial for this product, which it is not. When writing office notes, I even leave out the hyphen but somehow do not think the company would mind since I recommend this drug to my patients in preference to other time-release niacin products.

time for a new series of tablets to just under an hour. (I tell my patients 50 minutes so we have a definite figure in mind.)

The new product's label shows the "EP" logo (the letters joined together, with an arrow as the top rung of the E). Then it says "plain niacin," which it is, by the FDA definition. On my charts and in my writing, I called this 50-minute product "EP NA;" in conversation, "EP plain niacin." I no longer use the old-fashioned, three- to five-minute NA, which we now call "unmodified" niacin to keep things straight. I have nothing against unmodified niacin, which has served us well since 1955; I just think EP NA is better.

By delaying dissolution and absorption by nearly an hour, EP NA seems to have the characteristics of the old. unmodified niacin (less nausea, less alteration in liver tests, greater increases in "good" HDLC) while largely eliminating any significant flush. We still advise the morning aspirin. Some persons feel some flushing an hour or so after taking this product, but it is seldom troublesome. When he first tried EP NA. one of my tennis colleagues, who was taking unmodified NA to raise his HDLC, said, "If the flush from the old one was a 10, this is a two." He later changed his appraisal to "a one."

In the late 1950's and the 1960's I worked with an intermediate-release niacin product, which was marketed in 1960 and withdrawn about 1980 (because of lack of profitability, as far as I know). Called aluminum nicotinate, or Nicalex, it delayed absorption perhaps 60 to 90 minutes, which was enough to prevent flushing. Used in my studies since before it was marketed, it showed an incidence of nausea and liver test alterations which was intermediate between NA and the TRNA preparations then available. At first I thought EP NA might share these characteristics of intermediate-release Nicalex, but to date this has not been the case.

When I first learned about EP NA, my instinctive feeling was that it was a major breakthrough, possibly the most significant development since the Canadians' suggestion reached me in 1955. The new product could be the answer to a niacin therapist's prayer for a product without flushing and also without the increased nausea and hepatic (liver) function abnormalities which occur in a minority of patients who use time-release preparations, even under proper supervision. My experience with the new product covers only a couple years at this writing, but so far nothing has happened to change this optimistic expectation.

Becoming Good At Niacin

In the following chapters I will explain how a physician can put into practice what I have learned about cholesterol control in more than forty years of experience. It will not hurt for readers without a medical degree also to have this information if they observe the warning repeated throughout this book: *Niacin is not a do-it-yourself drug. It must be taken under knowledgeable medical supervision.*

CHAPTER SIX

Starting Treatment and Adjusting Dosage with Plain or Time-Release Niacin

A Quick Review

In my Mayo Clinic study and early Madison studies, we used the starting dose of plain niacin (NA) suggested by the Canadians, 1000 mg three times a day, taken with meals. The Coronary Drug Project (CDP) also used this dose but reached it by two stepwise increases. My studies in Madison showed that more than half of patients required higher doses, but the CDP did not exceed 3000 mg per day.

Time-release niacin (TRNA) must be given in lower dosage, usually about half that of NA, since *the effect of TRNA is approximately twice that of NA, mg for mg.* Failure to observe this rule could cause serious problems, notably toxic effects on the liver, discussed later. This is the main reason that use of niacin requires knowledgeable medical supervision, as opposed to self-administration by patients. If a patient were to switch from NA to TRNA in the same dosage, the consequences could be very serious. Before starting treatment, each patient receives my sheets of information for those who are going to take niacin (Appendix A).

There are differences in the absorption characteristics of various time-release preparations. As already pointed out, I advise each doctor to choose one or two products and insist that patients use only those preparations.

Regardless of the type of niacin, I have a patient take one 325 mg aspirin tablet (the usual adult size) immediately on arising in the morning, swallowing it with six to eight ounces of water. Although flushing is merely a nuisance effect, patients are more comfortable if we minimize it early in treatment. Later each person can decide whether continuing aspirin is necessary.

Starting Time-Release Niacin (TRNA)

I usually start niacin in time-release form. This eliminates most symptoms related to flushing, especially with the morning aspirin. Using only 500 mg caplets of TRNA allows me to talk with patients in terms of *how many* caplets they are taking, without having to specify the strength. (For the same reason, I use only 500 mg tablets of plain niacin.)

Customarily I have a patient take *one TRNA caplet daily* for the *first week,* usually with breakfast. In the *second week* I increase the dose to one caplet *twice a* day, at breakfast and supper. If all is going well, in the *third week* I usually increase the dose to one caplet *three times a day.* Doses may be taken with meals, but TRNA may be taken on an empty stomach without ill effects. This dose, one 500 mg caplet three times a day, continues until the end of four weeks, when we recheck the lipid profile (total cholesterol, plus LDLC and HDLC fractions) and see the patient.

If any problem should occur, the patient knows to *call me.* This is especially important if there should be troublesome side effects. I instruct patients *never* to stop the drug and tell me this on the next office visit. Usually by telephone I can help the patient over problems with side effects, based on my long experience with niacin—longer, after all, than anyone else in the world. Any doctor who becomes good at niacin can do the same.

If I have doubts about the patient's ability to handle two dosage increases in the first month, I leave the dose at two caplets instead of increasing to 500 mg three times a day after the second week. In such instances, I mention that the lipid fractions will probably not be in the desirable ranges after four weeks, although some persons (probably less than 10%) need only 500 mg twice a day for proper control. I make sure the patient knows that *the average dose of TRNA is three to four caplets a day* (1500 to 2000 mg a day), with some patients needing more (five or six caplets, a total of 2500 or 3000 mg a day).

After the First Month

If lipid values are in the desirable ranges after four weeks, with both the bad (LDL) and good (HDL) cholesterol in desirable ranges, we continue the successful dose. When results are borderline, it may be a good idea to recheck the lipids after another four or eight weeks to be sure the favorable effects are stable. Since they almost always will be, I more often go right to a twelve-week follow-up interval.

If we are going to wait twelve weeks before seeing the patient again, I phone the laboratory and have them perform a *liver profile* on frozen serum saved from the just-repeated lipid profile. Otherwise, I include the liver profile along with the lipids the next time, in four or eight weeks. The basic principle is this: when we have reached the correct dose for proper cholesterol control, liver function should be assessed so the physician will know the hepatic (liver) enzyme levels at this dose. The results of the liver tests will usually be entirely normal. If there should be *mild elevations* in one or more of the enzymes, these have *no clinical significance.*

You have just read one of the most important sentences in this book! It is my guess that the most common error by physicians who are not good at niacin is to stop the drug because of *minor elevations* in liver enzymes that are actually *a normal part of niacin therapy.* These minor elevations occur in a minority of patients and have no significance; however, it is best for the doctor to know about the mild changes so neither he nor any other doctor seeing the patient will think something other than niacin causes them. Only if the levels reach two to three times the upper limit of normal or are accompanied by nausea does it become prudent to discontinue niacin, at least temporarily. More detail in this regard is in Chapter 7, *Side Effects of Niacin and Their Management.*

Another important point: *Whatever dose was necessary to achieve desirable levels will usually be the dose needed to maintain this improvement.* If a cholesterol control drug is stopped, the body factory will return lipid levels to their pre-treatment ranges quite soon. Trying to maintain improvement with reduced doses has not been successful.

If lipid levels are not yet in the desirable ranges after the first month, further treatment decisions depend on their levels and how the patient feels. Table 8 is an algorithm summarizing the usual recommendations for dosage changes at monthly intervals, depending on whether LDLC and/or HDLC have reached target levels or are still out of line.

At four weeks, the patient should be tolerating 500 mg of TRNA three times a day. If the cholesterol fractions are not in the desirable ranges, the dose should be increased to *four caplets a day* for the next four weeks. These may be taken in any pattern, just so they are not taken all at once. (A brief early trial in Madison showed that taking all the niacin as a single daily dose did not reduce cholesterol as well.) A patient may take one caplet four times a day, or she may choose to take one at breakfast and lunch, then two at supper. A busy working person who has trouble remembering a noon dose may elect to take two caplets twice a day. Any of these schedules seems to be effective, so convenience and tolerance should be the deciding factors.

Even on average doses, a patient may, although not really nauseated, feel slightly queasy part of the time. After assessing the severity of this discomfort, I often tell the patient to omit the final caplet on such days. The symptom, usually mild and not present every day, can ordinarily be handled

Table 8

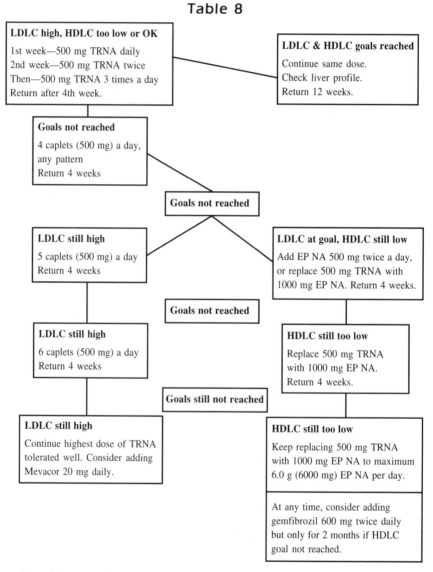

Algorithm for adjusting dosage of time-release niacin (TRNA)

successfully in this manner while still achieving good lipid control. On the next visit I ask the patient to estimate the percentage of days on full dosage. If she has taken four tablets on 60% of days and three the rest of the time, we record the average daily dose as 3.6 caplets.

Before mentioning several cases that show how I adjusted dosage, let's review the goals of treatment. NCEP calls total cholesterol (*TC*) "desirable" if *below 200*, but we have already seen that TC can be misleading unless one knows both bad and good cholesterol levels. For *LDL* (bad) cholesterol, the target is *below 100* for anyone with a previous cardiovascular event, *below 130* for everyone else—even though NCEP permits *less than 160* as a target with fewer than two risk factors. We want to see *HDL* (good) cholesterol *above 45* but sometimes have to settle for levels between 40 and 45.

A typical case showing good control of cholesterol at the end of the first month with 500 mg of Endur-acin three times a day (Table 9) was a 46-year-old auto service advisor with no clinical coronary disease or other arterial events. His TC fell from its pre-treatment average of 249 (266, 242) to 193, LDLC from 180 (190, 160) to 128. These are satisfactory levels for a man without known vascular disease, so we checked his liver tests (normal), continued the successful dose, and had him return twelve weeks later with another lipid profile. HDLC levels were in the high 40's to mid-50's, before and after treatment.

Table 9
Success on Three Caplets a Day
46 M, auto service advisor

Date	Treatment	Cholesterol	LDLC	HDLC
2-28	0	266	190	56
3-27	0	242	169	53
4-21	Endur-acin 1.5 g/day	193	128	46

To show that older persons tolerate TRNA as well as their younger counterparts, Table 10 shows success on three caplets a day in an 82-year-old woman, a retired school principal with very good general health and a delightfully sharp mind. Her pre-treatment average TC of 258 (253, 262) fell to 210 and LDLC from 173 to 107. HDLC, already in a good range (average 70 before treatment), rose to 96. This illustrates the situation in which HDLC may be so high that TC is above the "desirable" limit of 200 and yet the pattern is ideal. Liver tests were normal. We had her return in 12 weeks.

Table 10
Success on Three Caplets per Day
82F, retired school principal

Date	Treatment	Cholesterol	LDLC	HDLC
2-7	0	253	163	78
2-24	0	262	183	62
3-25	Endur-acin 1.5 g/day	210	107	96

After the Second Month

If lipid fractions are now in desirable ranges. I have the laboratory perform liver tests, as outlined above. Then the proper interval for further follow-up, with lipid testing and an office visit, is 12 weeks. *This interval remains the same as long as treatment continues.* If the dosage remains stable and the patient feels good, I am comfortable rechecking liver tests only with annual examinations, but the physician should individualize this according to his comfort level. The 12-week interval should begin when the lipid levels are satisfactory, regardless of when this occurs. I will not repeat "if lipid levels are in the desirable range" after this.

After any adjustment in the niacin dose, the patient should return for lipid testing and an office visit four weeks later. This principle also continues throughout treatment.

If lipid values are still not in desirable ranges. with LDLC still too high and if nausea is not a problem, I increase TRNA to *five caplets (total 2500 mg) per day*, in any pattern except all at once. I make sure the patient understands that we tend to encounter nausea more frequently on five or six caplets a day than on lower doses. However, this should not deter using the higher doses if patients tolerate them without symptoms.

A 51-year-old nurse aide came to me with hypercholesteremia and obesity. She had no known cardiovascular disease, but her father had had a heart attack at age 54 and her mother was diabetic. She had been taking a statin (Pravachol), which had not provided adequate control of her cholesterol problem (Table 11). Her TC was 288, with LDLC of 208. HDLC was satisfactory at 60. Her weight was 165, too much for a short woman. We stopped her Pravachol and decided to see whether weight reduction might reduce her cholesterol levels. Six months later she had lost 11 pounds but remained heavy. TC was 330, LDLC 237; HDLC was 66.

Table 11
Success on Five Caplets per Day
51F, nurse aide

Date	Treatment	Cholesterol	LDLC	HDLC
7-31	0	288	208	60
1-14	0	330	237	66
2-21	Endur-acin 1.5 g/day	317	195	68
3-21	Endur-acin 2.0 g/day	286	197	59
4-18	Endur-acin 2.5 g/day	217	126	77

Starting Endur-acin with the 1-2-3 caplet plan over the first few weeks reduced LDLC from 237 only to 195 and TC from 330 only to 317, not satisfactory levels. Increasing the dose to four caplets a day reduced TC to 286, but LDLC remained at 197. Adding a fifth caplet daily reduced these values, as shown in the table, to TC 217 with LDLC 126; this dose also raised her HDLC to 77. Liver tests gave normal results. We scheduled her next lipid profile and office visit 12 weeks later.

If, after the second month, LDLC is satisfactory but *HDLC is too low*, I now *add EP NA* 500 mg twice a day or *replace* one 500 mg caplet of TRNA with 1000 mg of EP NA. The reason: plain niacin has been found (two reports, plus my own experience) to be more effective in raising HDLC than TRNA. The converse appears to be true: TRNA is slightly more effective at reducing LDLC than plain niacin. However, either type of niacin does both (reduces LDLC and increases HDLC). Giving each of them credit for doing one thing slightly better than the other is almost splitting hairs. Nevertheless, this distinction serves the doctor well as he plans therapy, especially in raising

HDLC. In subsequent months, it may be necessary to add more EP NA if HDLC is stubborn.

I do not always add EP NA when the patient is tolerating TRNA well and the HDLC "good" cholesterol needs more help. In 1993 a 72-year-old house painter came to me with cholesterol and vascular problems. He had had a coronary artery bypass procedure in 1982 and had lost his left leg above the knee from arterial impairment in 1992. After performing a balloon angioplasty on the right femoral artery in 1993, his vascular surgeon had told him the circulation was bad in the remaining leg and he could do nothing more for him. Such a gloomy outlook understandably depressed the gentleman. I explained that the surgeon meant that he could do nothing more for him *surgically*, but we would take use medical measures known to retard new cholesterol deposits and possibly reduce some existing plaques.

Table 12 shows some of the painter's cholesterol values. TC was 171 before treatment and 162 after one month on TRNA 500 mg twice a day. LDLC was 108, 103 and HDLC 37, 43. After a month of 500 mg three times a day, the levels were about the same. EP NA was not available in those days. I increased his TRNA to four caplets a day, which reduced LDLC to 82 and increased HDLC to 52. The TC was 152, not much of a drop because good cholesterol rose as bad cholesterol fell. I have previously mentioned this situation, which made cholesterol results in the early days of niacin look less impressive than they would have been if LDLC and HDLC fractions had been measured instead of just the TC.

In 1997, about four years after first coming to my office, this painter is still climbing up and down ladders. He now takes Endur-acin 500 mg three times a day. Recent LDLC levels have been 86 and 97, HDLC 63 and 52, TC 158 and 162. His spirits are much better than right after his surgeon's dismal forecast in 1993.

What is the maximum dose of unmodified NA or EP NA? No one really knows. In the early years, when we had only plain niacin, I increased the initial dose of 3000 mg a day to 4500 mg and to 6000 mg to achieve better control in the first few months. Sometimes I increased the dosage further to 7500 or 9000 mg a day for many months, sometimes a year or longer. (Although we determined bad and good cholesterol fractions in those days, we governed treatment by the total cholesterol level.) One evening I sat and listed on spreadsheets the results in patients who had received more than 6000 mg (6.0 g) per day. The results didn't improve on doses higher than 6.0 g a day, so thereafter my writings said that there was no reason to exceed that level.

Table 12
Success on Three to Four Caplets
72M. house painter

Date	Treatment	Cholesterol	LDLC	HDLC
9-8 -93	0	171	108	37
10-4	TRNA 1.0 g/day	162	103	43
11-2	TRNA 1.5 g/day	167	101	46
11-30	TRNA 2.0 g/day	152	82	52
3-1-94	Same	162	96	46
(Treatment continued with similar results)				
2-26-97	Endur-acin 1.5 g/day	158	86	63
4-14	Same	162	97	52

There's always an exception that proves the rule. Years later, in Scottsdale, a woman's cholesterol level had remained elevated on 6.0 g of plain niacin each day. I told her this story about doses above that level, but she said, "Why don't we try and see?" Having comfortably used 7.5 g or even 9.0 g a day in many patients during the early Madison years, I agreed to such a trial. The 7.5 mg a day dose satisfactorily controlled her cholesterol factory. Let me re-emphasize that such sizeable doses apply only to *plain niacin* (EP NA or unmodified NA). Using TRNA doses larger than 3.0 g (six 500 mg caplets) a day is risky, and I do not exceed this level.

If it is necessary to increase plain niacin to higher levels for HDLC control, it may be best to replace TRNA entirely, using two 500 mg tablets of NA or EP NA to replace each 500 mg caplet of TRNA. Thus a patient who had been on four TRNA caplets would be changed to eight 500 mg tablets of EP NA, which is less likely to cause nausea or alter liver function tests. I would have no problem with increasing the EP NA dose to as much as 9.0 g (9000 mg, 18 tablets) a day, based on prior experience with unmodified NA. However, I have not found this to be necessary in two decades in Scottsdale, probably because most of my current patients receive one of the excellent time-release products now available.

In Subsequent Months

If LDLC is still too high on five 500 mg caplets of TRNA and nausea is not a problem, I increase to *six caplets a day*, again warning the patient that more nausea occurs at higher doses. If six caplets a day (usually 1000 mg three times) fails to control LDLC after another four weeks and HDLC is satisfactory, I consider *adding 20 mg of Mevacor daily* and recheck a month later. Before adding this "statin," I check liver tests to be sure all is well on niacin alone. I am not aware that this combination has caused more liver test abnormalities than either drug alone, but since both have this potential, it is best to be sure. There is a slight increase in percentage risk of the muscle problems ("myopathy") caused by Mevacor when combined with niacin (about 2% of patients), so the doctor-patient team should watch for this possibility. (For details, see Chapter 8, *The Other Drugs for Cholesterol Control.*)

If HDLC is still too low (not above 45) after we have replaced TRNA with EP NA (or unmodified niacin, which I no longer use) to full dosage (6.0 g a day), *I add gemfibrozil (Lopid)*. Although reputed to increase HDLC, this drug has been inconsistent in my experience. ("Disappointing" is a better word.) If its usual dose, 600 mg twice a day, fails to produce the desired HDLC level in two months, *discontinue gemfibrozil*, in keeping with FDA's instructions. Using this drug with niacin has not caused any difficulty.

Even before the NCEP advised (1993) keeping HDLC out of the danger zone below 35, I was using the PSG (Parsons Simplified Guidelines) and keeping this value above 45. By using HDLC as one criterion for adjusting dosage, I learned a lesson which should be shared with doctors supervising niacin therapy. Unlike LDLC and TC, which fell dramatically in the first week on niacin when I started using the drug in Rochester, HDLC may take longer to rise to desirable levels. So if, after the first month, LDLC is well controlled and HDLC is moving toward the desired above-45 level, more aggressive measures to raise HDLC may not be needed. I usually wait another month for HDLC to increase further. If it fails to do so, one of the adjustments to improve it, mentioned above, is warranted.

If TC and LDLC are "too low." Too low? Isn't it desirable to have the bad cholesterol (and thus the total) as low as possible? *Not always.* Cholesterol is needed in the body, as a component of cell walls and a necessary ingredient in production of adrenal hormones and sex hormones. Some reports have suggested that pushing cholesterol "too low" might have led to adverse events, including more deaths from cancer, accidents, and suicides. Today the best informed analysis of the situation says that the low cholesterol levels were the result, not the cause, of cancer and other serious conditions. Low cholesterol levels do not result in psychiatric difficulties leading to accidents and suicides.

Nevertheless, in my experience, there is good reason to adjust dosage if total cholesterol is "too low" (125 or lower), with correspondingly low LDLC. For some reason, in this situation the HDLC, which niacin usually increases, may also be below the desirable range. The proper action is to reduce the niacin dose and recheck a month later, by which time the values will probably be satisfactory.

How long to continue niacin? Despite my printed information, a patient occasionally asks how long it will be necessary to continue taking niacin (or any drug for cholesterol control). My answer: as long as you want to control the cholesterol pattern to prevent heart attacks and strokes. The body factory will resume its old, nasty habits if we discontinue treatment.

Is this always this the case? Can the body factory change its tune and not require control by medication? Not as a rule, but I have occasionally seen this happen. In the Madison days, sometimes we completed a study of a cholesterol-lowering agent, and needed to get patients ready for the next study. We customarily stopped active medication, and substituted a placebo (a blank tablet or capsule resembling an active drug) for eight to twelve weeks before the next program. In this way, the patient served as his own control, and we did not have to give placebo to half of our participants throughout a study. In a very few persons the cholesterol levels did not return to an abnormal range. We then informed the patient and continued to observe without treatment. Most levels eventually rose again, but very rarely they did not.

One might expect that if major metabolic changes occur, the body factory for cholesterol might change. Loss of a large amount of weight or improved control of diabetes can theoretically change the body factory. In my experience this seldom happens. We ordinarily have diabetes under good control before starting a cholesterol-control drug. One situation which can cause hypercholesteremia and should be normalized before using such a drug is *low thyroid function (hypothyroidism)*. Our test for hypothyroidism (serum TSH, which stands for <u>th</u>yroid-<u>s</u>timulating <u>h</u>ormone) is so good at detecting even minor degrees of thyroid deficiency that we seldom encounter severe hypothyroidism today. The TSH test should always precede specific cholesterol treatment. If needed, proper replacement by the correct dose of synthetic thyroid tablets should be in place before measuring baseline cholesterol readings.

If a patient has been on niacin or any of the other drugs for a long time and the doctor wants to see whether the body factory still needs to be adjusted, there's nothing wrong with a month's drug holiday to let cholesterol levels drift back to baseline. They will undoubtedly return to their former levels, showing that ongoing treatment is needed. I rarely use this strategy but would do so if a patient were to request it. This maneuver would require a one-month recheck when we have been sailing along at comfortable 12-week intervals, so we usually leave well enough alone.

Starting Plain Niacin

Even though I have stated my preference for TRNA to initiate treatment and explained that such preparations are easily managed by a doctor good at niacin, there will be some who still believe assertions that TRNA causes liver toxicity and only plain niacin should be used. This section is to help anyone who chooses to begin treatment with a plain niacin preparation instead of TRNA, which I use. I am comfortable outlining how this is done; after all, originally we had nothing except unmodified niacin.

Let's remember that there are now two types of plain (dissolves in less than one hour) niacin: unmodified niacin (NA), which dissolves in three to five minutes, and EP NA, which takes about 50 minutes to dissolve. Each has the advantage of tending to cause less nausea and less alteration in hepatic (liver) function tests than equivalent doses of TRNA. Equivalent doses would be approximately twice as many mg for NA or EP NA as for TRNA, because of the latter's greater action on lipids.

I see no reason to start NA or EP NA in doses less than we used in the late 1950's, *1000 mg three times a day*, with meals. As previously explained, this results in rapid reduction of flushing in the first several days, with its disappearance (for all practical purposes) in an average of three to four days. Starting with low doses and increasing gradually is the best way I know to prolong the flush, and yet this is what today's medical literature recommends. All authors seem to copy from the papers of others, thinking this to be the politically correct method. They should be copying my papers of the late 1950's, my chapters in the Altschul and Casdorph books, and writings by my former Mayo colleagues and other investigators of that era.

Ungrammatically, I call the modern pussyfooting approach the "start low, go slow" method. At least this prevalent concept only wastes time; it does not deprive anyone of niacin therapy as the earlier-mentioned error, discontinuing the drug because of slight increases in hepatic enzymes.

Giving the patient printed information (Appendix A) to read before using niacin will often lead to smoother acceptance of the temporary inconvenience of short-term flushing. Plain niacin should be taken with meals, preferably mid-meal or just after eating. The morning aspirin trick is essential. As with TRNA, the lipid profile should be rechecked and the patient seen after four weeks. Some patients call sooner to complain about the flush, especially on the first day, sometimes after only one dose. The physician good at niacin uses this opportunity to remind the patient that the flush will subside and soon not be a problem. Re-reading the pre-treatment information about niacin will remind the patient of its reassuring message.

Adjustment of dosage for plain niacin consists of increasing the dose to a more effective level if both LDLC and HDLC are not in desirable ranges by the end of the first month, the second month, or after that. If 1000 mg three times a day fails to provide proper control, I would increase to *1500 mg three times a day*, always with meals. If this fails to reach goals in another month, increase to *2000 mg three times a day*. Remember that increasing the dose *does not* cause further flushing.

If this should not reduce LDLC satisfactorily, I would probably change to TRNA—but what dose to use? Rather than use the approximate equivalent, which would be 1000 mg (two 500 mg caplets) three times a day, it is better to use only three or four 500 mg caplets of TRNA each day and adjust from there.

If LDLC is satisfactory but HDLC is too low, the doctor will decide whether to wait another month for the slower-than-LDLC response, as already discussed, or to increase the dose of plain niacin, the most effective agent for raising HDLC.

Certain principles remain the same for NA or EP NA as for TRNA follow-up. Once we reach satisfactory levels of bad and good cholesterol fractions, the follow-up intervals to recheck lipids and an office visit may be increased to 12 weeks. The liver tests should be done when the right dose of NA is reached, then repeated at whatever interval the physician finds comfortable. For me it is at annual examinations, unless the patient develops nausea or anything else to suggest hepatitis along the way. (It really isn't hepatitis, but some authors like to call it that in the medical literature, and I'm not going to quarrel about such a small point.) If adjustment of the dose becomes necessary, lipid values should be checked a month later and the patient advised further.

A Final Reminder

No doctor should have trouble following these patterns for starting either type of niacin and adjusting doses according to the response of the cholesterol fractions. Those who have never used niacin because of a bias fostered by niacin detractors will quickly develop confidence in its use. So will those who may have dabbled in its use without the solid background they have received by reading this book. The next chapter on how to manage possible side effects should bolster that confidence. It also lists the few situations that make it advisable to stop niacin and use a different type of drug. A subsequent chapter on the other drugs (Chapter 8) will offer further guidance in this regard, as will further details in the medical section.

Don't ever forget: *Niacin is not a do-it-yourself drug. It requires knowledgeable medical supervision.*

Summary

◆ The flushing characteristic of old-fashioned, unmodified niacin (NA) can be prevented by taking a single 325 mg aspirin tablet each morning and starting treatment with time-release niacin (TRNA).

◆ Using only 500 mg caplets or tablets of niacin, regardless of the type of niacin preparation the doctor chooses, improves communication between patient and physician, who can talk about "How many tablets?" without having to ask "What strength?"

◆ Starting with one caplet a day and increasing to two and to three caplets at weekly intervals is a convenient regimen for most patients. If LDL (bad) cholesterol is not adequately controlled, the dose may be increased at monthly intervals to four, five, or six caplets if nausea does not interfere.

◆ A patient who feels queasy at times may omit the final caplet on those days and thus tolerate an intermediate dose. Real nausea, if it subsides without niacin but recurs each time the drug is used at the needed dose, requires that the drug be stopped.

◆ When therapist and patient have found the dose that controls LDLC and HDLC to target levels, liver tests (at least the enzymes SGOT and SGPT— also called ALT and AST) should be performed. Minor elevations in these enzymes are a part of niacin therapy in some patients and need not interrupt the program. Enzyme elevations two to three times higher than the upper limits of normal, often accompanied by nausea and other symptoms simulating hepatitis, require that niacin be discontinued. The enzyme levels promptly return to normal (usually within one week, two at most) and symptoms subside.

◆ A patient who discontinues TRNA because of nausea and/or liver dysfunction may be able to tolerate a plain niacin preparation, which causes these side effects in fewer persons.

◆ Endurance Products Plain Niacin (EP NA), a relatively new product, usually eliminates flushing because it takes 50 minutes to dissolve (compared to the very rapid dissolution time of unmodified niacin, three to five minutes). It appears to have the benefits of plain niacin (less nausea and alteration of liver function tests) without significant flushing.

◆ If one chooses to start therapy with plain niacin, either unmodified (NA) or EP NA, whatever flush occurs will subside sooner if the starting dose is 1000 mg three times a day, with meals. Starting lower and increasing more slowly prolongs the flush and wastes time. The morning aspirin trick should always be used when starting plain niacin.

◆ Increases of plain niacin from a total of 3000 mg a day to 4500 mg or 6000 mg a day, as used in the early days, are reasonable and can be recommended with impunity. Doses of 7500 mg or 9000 mg a day usually (but not invariably) fail to control cholesterol levels better than a total of 6000 mg a day. Because of its intermediate-release pattern, EP NA may not require such large stepwise increases.

◆ In general, plain niacin preparations (NA, EP NA) are more effective at raising HDL (good) cholesterol than TRNA. On the other hand, TRNA may be more effective in reducing LDLC than plain niacin. However, regardless of its absorption pattern, every niacin product effects favorable changes in both LDLC and HDLC fractions, as well as their subfractions, including Lp(a).

◆ If HDLC remains too low after TRNA satisfactorily controls LDLC, the physician may choose to add EP NA or replace part of the TRNA with equivalent amounts of plain niacin.

◆ As a rule of thumb, TRNA is about twice as effective, mg for mg, as plain niacin. It is, therefore, vitally important that TRNA *never* be substituted for NA or EP NA in the same mg dosage. Serious, even fatal, consequences have followed such a mistake. (See Medical Section.)

◆ If well-tolerated doses of niacin do not control LDLC well, the physician may need to add another drug, usually a statin. If niacin preparations do not bring low HDLC levels to the desirable range, adding gemfibrozil may do so, but this drug should not be continued beyond two months if its use does not achieve the goal.

CHAPTER SEVEN

Side Effects of Niacin and Their Management

Both patient and physician need to know how to recognize and manage niacin's relatively few side effects. The doctor must be good at niacin and the patient must know that his physician is adept in its use. My reviewing this information in a book for patients does not change the truth I have already emphasized: Niacin is not a do-it-yourself drug. It requires knowledgeable medical supervision.

Cutaneous Flush

Flushing of the skin from plain niacin (NA) and time-release niacin (TRNA) and its management has already been thoroughly discussed in the chapters concerning the important differences between these products, how to start either type of niacin, and how to adjust their dosage.

Gastrointestinal Side Effects

Regarding gastrointestinal (stomach and intestinal) symptoms, my first Mayo report (May 1956) mentioned occasional occurrence of nausea during use of niacin in cholesterol-lowering doses. After describing flushing, (itching), and transient urticaria (hives), the account read, "Nausea was occasionally troublesome and because of it [the] study of two patients was discontinued in the early stages; one of these patients had experienced similar difficulty with other oral medication. One patient...had both nausea and urticaria [hives], but neither side effect recurred when treatment was resumed after it had been discontinued for two weeks." Nothing more was said about nausea in the 14-page paper that introduced the new method of treatment to the medical world.

My later reports from Madison reiterated that nausea and vomiting, although infrequent, caused enough discomfort in a few patients to stop the drug. When we tried time-release products from several manufacturers, who hoped to reduce flushing and have a patentable product, we encountered more nausea.

Remember that today's TRNA preparations have approximately twice the effect on lipids as NA, mg for mg. Therefore, for the same cholesterol-lowering effect, an equivalent dose of TRNA would be about half that of NA. Even in equivalent doses (TRNA half that of NA), TRNA causes a little more nausea and/or altered liver function tests. This does not mean that physicians should not prescribe TRNA; I have already pointed out that I usually start every new patient on this type of preparation. It just means that the doctor should be aware of this tendency as he supervises therapy.

If a patient reports nausea, with or without vomiting, while taking any form of niacin, I usually advise her to omit the drug for a week, then resume the previous dose. If stomach upset was due to another cause, such as food poisoning or viral gastroenteritis, it subsides, permitting continuation of niacin therapy. If nausea recurs, niacin was probably the cause.

At this point, one can still continue niacin therapy. Replacing TRNA with NA (including EP NA, which I would now use) and adjusting to the best dose will often work. Or the therapist could reduce the TRNA dose to a lower level, which has been tolerated without nausea. If the lower dose previously failed to produce the desired levels of cholesterol fractions, the same result will probably occur now. In this situation, continuing the reduced TRNA dose and adding NA or EP NA is worth trying.

In recent years a more common gastrointestinal side effect has been a queasy feeling, which does not interfere with treatment. In Chapter 6 I mentioned managing this by omitting the final caplet on any given day. This often accomplishes our goals without changing preparations.

Does niacin cause or activate peptic ulcer? *It does not.* However, this possibility is mentioned in FDA labeling, as well as in lists of side effects in anything written in the past few decades by niacin's detractors or others who just copy the list from everyone else.

Here's the true story. In 1960 I published a paper titled *Activation of Peptic Ulcer by Nicotinic Acid: Report of Five Cases.* In an addendum written after submission but before publication, I added two more case reports. More than three decades of experience since that article have taught me the truth about that paper: *It was wrong!*

Even in the paper itself, I expressed reservations that niacin was actually responsible for activating peptic ulcer, although the possibility did exist. Being young and feeling the responsibility of having introduced an important new method of therapy, I thought it best to publish my observations, alerting doctors and thus preventing possible harm to patients. My case reports even mentioned sources of great personal stress in nearly every patient who had active ulcers during niacin therapy. With one exception, every one of them had a prior history of ulcer, a scarred duodenum by x-ray (indicating a healed ulcer), or a history of significant gastrointestinal symptoms before using niacin.

How do I know that my 1960 paper was wrong and that warnings regarding ulcer activation are inappropriate? Since writing that paper, I have not seen a single case of active peptic ulcer in a patient taking niacin for hypercholesteremia. Furthermore, the CDP, which followed about 1,100 men on niacin and more than 2,700 men on placebo for five to eight years, did not report activation of ulcer. As expected, gastric symptoms were somewhat more frequent in the niacin group but no greater than already reported in the literature. The CDP reported decreased appetite in 4.27% of men on niacin (1.5% on placebo), nausea without vomiting in 8.5% (vs. 6.2%.), vomiting in 2.07% (1.3%), stomach pain in 13.9% (7.9%).

Do these seem like fairly high percentages of patients with each of these symptoms? They are not, because they represent percentages of CDP patients who complained of these side effects *at any time* (even once!) during five to eight years of follow-up. Considering this, the numbers are not at all impressive. To me, the most significant fact is that my 37 years of further experience (since my 1960 paper) and the CDP experience failed to demonstrate any cases in which the drug activated peptic ulcer. *My 1960 report regarding activation of peptic ulcers by niacin was wrong!*

What did others report about gastrointestinal (GI) symptoms and possible ulcer occurrence in the early days? In 1961 my former Mayo colleagues reviewed their experience in 66 patients, four of whom had discontinued treatment because of GI symptoms, usually loss of appetite or nausea. Responding to my ulcer report, they pointed out that they had found no instances of peptic ulcer and that two patients with previous ulcers had no aggravation of their symptoms. They later reported GI symptoms in 25 of 40 patients on the early TRNA preparations, none of which was ever marketed, but only one of 28 patients on plain niacin.

Does niacin cause diarrhea? The answer is "very infrequently." I have seen one patient discontinue the drug for this reason in my Scottsdale practice (since 1978). During my 18 years in Madison, there may have been a few persons with diarrhea, but it was not prominent and did not interfere with treatment. For diarrhea, the CDP listed a cumulative five-year total of only 4.6% of niacin participants *ever complaining of diarrhea* (on even one occasion), compared to 3.5% on placebo, an unimpressive difference. This means that the few participants who ever complained of diarrhea probably experienced it from other causes, not niacin.

What about gallstones, caused by one of the other types of drugs for cholesterol control? Niacin has not caused any increase in gallstones or in gall bladder surgery.

To be good at niacin, a physician needs to know how to adjust the dosage or type of preparation if nausea, with or without vomiting, should occur. If the adjustments outlined previously do not solve the problem while achieving the goals of treatment, there are two choices. One is to stop niacin and use a different agent, even though none of the others has niacin's distinctive advantages. The other is to use whatever niacin dose the patient tolerates and add a second drug if necessary to reach the goals of treatment. Perhaps in this way the doses of each drug can be kept relatively low, as with combinations of drugs for high blood pressure.

Nausea with vomiting can be associated with abnormalities in liver function which make it desirable to discontinue niacin, at least temporarily. Therefore, these symptoms can sometimes be a signal to check hepatic function tests and handle any abnormality properly, as outlined in the next section.

Changes in Hepatic Function Tests

When we first studied niacin, the automated chemical testing used in the past few decades had not yet been developed. Laboratory tests were ordered individually and performed manually, not by machines. We followed blood counts, kidney function tests, and the few hepatic (liver) function studies then available. At that time the best test of liver function involved an injection into a vein, then testing blood drawn from another vein 45 minutes later. In the 1960's this test was replaced by enzyme tests of hepatic function, which were adaptable to the new automated test batteries.

At first we found no significant abnormality in liver function tests during niacin therapy. After the first 18 patients had completed one year in my

Madison studies, I offered each of them a day in the hospital and a needle biopsy of the liver by one of our surgeons. Looking back, I find it hard to believe that I was so young and brash as to make this suggestion just because we needed the information. Even more incredibly, all except one of those patients agreed and had the biopsies performed. Two pathologists reviewed the slides and found *normal liver tissue* in every instance. This was very reassuring to me as a young investigator, still exploring uncharted ground.

After the first couple of years, both my participants and the Mayo Clinic patients receiving niacin began to show occasional abnormalities in hepatic function tests, mainly in the injection (BSP) test, which we followed periodically. Pioneering a new method of treatment puts one in a peculiar position. When questions arise, there is no one to ask who has more experience than you do. I compared notes periodically with Dick Achor and Ken Berge in Rochester. Together we tried to deduce the reason for the hepatic function abnormalities.

Our first thought was that the study patients had now been on niacin for about two years and perhaps toxic effects were appearing because of this duration of exposure. However, there was another possibility. By that time several pharmaceutical companies had developed delayed-release preparations and made them available for our studies. I must have used about ten such preparations over several years; the Mayo group used about three, including one I never had. Although it was not immediately apparent, we soon recognized that the abnormal hepatic function tests were occurring in persons receiving TRNA products. One product made this relationship especially obvious since it frequently caused nausea, along with the altered liver tests. When the drug was stopped, nausea promptly cleared and the considerably abnormal test results rapidly returned to normal.

I carefully studied the behavior of the abnormal liver function tests after discontinuing TRNA preparations. Before stopping the drug, we would verify the abnormal tests a week or two later. (The injection test could not be repeated sooner than a week later.) Then, after omitting the TRNA product, we would repeat liver tests two weeks later. *In every instance the results had returned to normal.* This was impressive. If tests had been this abnormal from alcoholic cirrhosis or liver damage from such toxins as benzene or carbon tetrachloride, we would have considered it fortunate for the results to return to normal in six months, even with the best of treatment.

After a while I tried repeating the tests only one week after stopping TRNA. *The results were normal.* Finally, I did not stop niacin at all; instead

I replaced the TRNA tablet with the *same dose of plain niacin*. Again the tests gave normal results a week later, making it clear that the delayed-release mechanism was causing the abnormal liver tests and the nausea as well.

The rapid return of hepatic function tests to normal, coupled with the uniformly normal needle biopsies in my 17 volunteers, convinced me that the abnormal results represented changes in liver *function* rather than actual anatomic *damage*. At that time it was difficult to get many physicians to understand this distinction. In contrast, over the years since then, FDA has approved numerous new drugs with an offhand statement that they may cause minor changes in hepatic function tests, which have no clinical significance. I believe my elucidation of this situation with niacin was the first demonstration that abnormal tests do not necessarily mean damage to hepatic cells with recognizable microscopic changes.

Rudolf Altschul, one of the Canadian originators of the niacin idea, compiled and edited a multi-author book on what was know about niacin in the early 1960's. I contributed a chapter titled *The Effect of Nicotinic Acid on the Liver: Evidence Favoring Functional Alteration of Enzymatic Reactions Without Hepatocelluler Damage*. Dr. Altschul's book, *Niacin in Vascular Disorders and Hyperlipemia*, was published in 1964. He had died a short time earlier while editing the book, which was completed by his associates at the University of Saskatchewan. This is not the place for a list of the facts on which I based my contention stated in the chapter title. I will include this list in this book's Medical Section.

The Coronary Drug Project (CDP) furnished the next demonstration of niacin's safety as regards the liver. Outlined previously, this study, (1966-1974) followed about 1,100 men receiving niacin for five to eight years. The study had an elaborate protocol to investigate significant alterations of hepatic function tests if any developed, including needle biopsies of the liver if needed. The results in periodic blood tests were shielded from investigators at the 53 clinical centers, mostly because the study was double-blind and we were not supposed to know which drug each patient was receiving. The reasoning was that we might identify niacin patients if we saw the mild changes in enzyme tests which are a normal part of niacin therapy in many. (Of course, those who flushed early in treatment were probably taking niacin, just as those with enlarged, tender breasts and loss of sexual potency were probably receiving Premarin.)

The results of the "hepatology protocol" were not specifically stated in the published account of the CDP results, so I asked the head statistician, Dr.

Paul Canner, about them. In a nutshell, the protocol had not been used very often. Its results, including liver biopsies when needed, showed *no abnormalities, which could be attributed to niacin* or, for that matter, any of the study drugs. In some instances there had been abnormal biopsy findings, but these were all due to alcohol, Canner assured me.

This discussion should reassure both the patient and the physician that it is all right to use niacin, especially those who may have been exposed to the flippant write-off of niacin (not only by niacin detractors, but also a prevalent incorrect rumor) that "The flush makes niacin hard to take, and it is toxic to the liver." Unfortunately, even among doctors who should be better informed, this undeserved derogatory bias has denied niacin's benefits to untold numbers of persons. This is another reason that every doctor should become knowledgeable about niacin and the patient should be trained to recognize the doctor who is.

To be good at niacin, a physician should first understand that most patients taking either NA or TRNA will have *normal* liver function results throughout treatment. Then he should remember that *minor elevations in enzyme tests reflecting liver function are a normal part of niacin therapy and are not a reason to discontinue treatment.* Minor elevations are those less than twice the upper limit of normal.

If the enzyme results *exceed two to three times the upper limit of normal*, the changes *are* significant and require *discontinuation of niacin*. Resuming later, either at a lower dosage or replacing TRNA with NA or EP NA is a subsequent option, but stopping the drug, at least temporarily, will let the test results return to normal. My Madison experience taught me that the results usually return to normal in one week, but I now recheck the laboratory studies two weeks after stopping the drug. Significant elevations of the liver function enzymes may be accompanied by nausea, often with vomiting. Some authors have called this "hepatitis" or "niacin hepatitis." As noted, it is rapidly reversible with proper management.

How often should liver tests be performed? As outlined in Chapter 6, I recommend performing the liver profile when the correct dose of niacin has been found. The medical section of this book details which tests are needed and which others to add if significant abnormalities appear. The results will almost always be normal. A few patients will show minor, insignificant elevations in one or more enzyme levels. If the niacin dosage then remains stable and the patient feels good, I am comfortable performing the tests only with annual examinations. For a doctor just developing confidence in handling niacin, one additional liver profile after six months, or halfway between the "correct dose" test and the next annual examination might be a good idea.

In 1996 I completed and copyrighted a manuscript much longer than this book, which presented abundant medical detail for physicians but in plain language, understandable to the nonmedical reader. (A helpful editor counseled me to write this book, aimed at the average reader but with a medical section adding useful details for doctors.) In the larger volume, a key chapter reviewed all reports of liver problems located in my search of the literature. The important fact to note here is that there were *only 18 cases reported*, with varying degrees of liver problems. Only a couple had serious, irreversible consequences. That's not bad for a drug used for more than 40 years, with more widespread use in recent years, much of it as a result of the NCEP guidelines of 1988 and 1993. Many of the cases showed that abnormal liver function was detected when the patient experienced symptoms and emphasized how promptly both the test results and the clinical problems resolved when the drug was stopped.

Further details will be found in the Medical Section of this book, which the nonmedical reader will have no trouble understanding. Several of the problems involved unwise changes from NA to TRNA in the same dosage, a danger which has already been discussed. In more than one case, the change was recommended by a pharmacist who obviously did not know the important distinction between the two types of products. A few others involved self-administration by patients or failure to follow medical advice regarding monitoring of laboratory tests.

Changes in Blood Glucose (Sugar)

In early studies (Madison, Rochester, various other centers) we found that niacin's use was often associated with increases in blood sugar (glucose), which are usually mild. Usually the increase is only 10 to 15 mg%, about the same as with commonly used diuretic medications; this does not interfere with therapy. The slight increase in glucose levels has no significance unless a doctor mistakes it for diabetes.

Ordinarily there is no problem with using niacin in diabetic patients *on diet alone* or *diet plus oral antidiabetic agents*. However, in *insulin-dependent diabetics*, I have seen niacin alter glucose levels enough to change the insulin requirements and make diabetic control erratic. Although I have given niacin to a few diabetics on insulin, especially in recent years, when home glucose testing makes monitoring easier, *I do not advise its use in such patients.*

In Madison (1957) a patient with very high cholesterol levels and hard lumps of cholesterol, called xanthomas, under the skin of his elbows and knees became a study patient. (We will discuss the skin lumps in another section.) Despite known vascular disease in his legs, he was applying for more life insurance and was notified that a urine sample sent to the home office had contained sugar. I contacted the company, explaining that the new form of treatment for hypercholesteremia was capable of raising blood glucose levels, possibly high enough to spill sugar in the urine. To resolve the uncertainty, I offered to stop treatment for only a week, recheck his blood glucose and urine glucose tests, and inform them of the results.

Somehow I knew from earlier experience that the changes in carbohydrate tolerance would subside promptly. The glucose levels after a week were entirely normal. We then resumed niacin without difficulty; if subsequent tests showed higher than normal blood sugar, this did not interfere with treatment. He did not ever become diabetic. Figure 2 shows how well his very high cholesterol level had been falling before the week's interruption of treatment. It rose abruptly when niacin was discontinued briefly, and fell again when we resumed the drug. These changes showed a marked abnormality in his body factory, as did the presence of the cholesterol deposits in the skin.

When a cortisone-like preparation such as prednisone is given to a latent diabetic (one who has inherited the disorder but in whom it has not yet become clinically evident), the diabetes will often appear and will persist after the cortisone-like preparation is stopped. Prednisone has "unmasked" the latent diabetes, which now is a permanent disorder. Niacin *does not* unmask latent diabetes. The changes in blood glucose due to niacin subside promptly if the drug is stopped, but this is not necessary since these changes have no adverse clinical consequences. A doctor good at niacin notices the relatively mild increases in glucose, does not mistake them for diabetes, and proceeds with treatment. If he should become uncertain about whether elevated levels of blood glucose are from niacin or diabetes, the question can be resolved by stopping niacin for a short time. If the changes are due to niacin, they promptly return to normal. If this does not happen, the patient has become diabetic. Niacin *did not* precipitate this condition.

Figure 2

Mr. G.H. (M, 46) Xanthoma Tuberosum, ASO

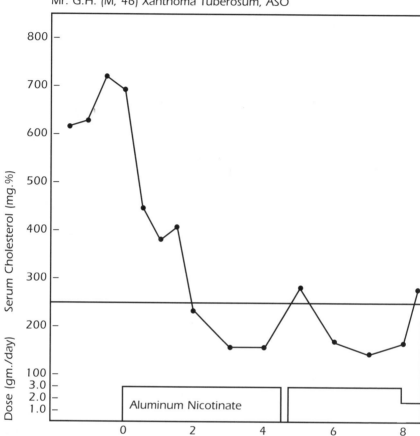

Graph of total cholesterol (TC) values for 46-year-old man with occlusive arterial disease in his legs ("ASO") and lumps of cholesterol under his skin of elbows and knees (xanthoma tuberosum). Some details of his clinical course are spelled out in the text. Before treatment with a niacin product (aluminum nicotinate), four cholesterol values were between 600 and 725. In two weeks the value fell sharply to 430. By the end of two months the cholesterol levels remained in the then-normal range, below 250, with two values at less than 150.

Between 4 and 5 months his insurance company found sugar in a urine specimen submitted when he applied for an additional policy. We stopped niacin for one week to show that the elevated blood sugar and urine sugar were related to niacin, not diabetes. During that week TC rose from less than 150 to more than 250. After resuming niacin, TC values were again between 100 and 150. Reducing the dose from 3.0 grams daily to 1.5 grams allowed the TC to exceed 250 again. Resuming the 3.0-gram dose (after the period shown on this graph) again controlled the TC to normal levels.

Changes in Uric Acid

As mentioned previously, laboratory tests were done manually and ordered individually when we first studied niacin. Nowadays a uric acid test is included in the usual multi-test chemistry battery, but in the 1950's it was not foremost in our thoughts, as were blood counts, liver and kidney function, and glucose. Nevertheless, before long we found that uric acid, like glucose, increased during treatment. In my chapter in a 1970 book (*Treatment of the Hyperlipidemic States*, edited by H. Richard Casdorph, M.D.), I summarized what was then known about niacin therapy, including uric acid results, from my work and that of the Mayo group. We agreed that uric acid increased somewhat during niacin therapy but that hyperuricemia (too much uric acid in the blood) should not interfere with ongoing treatment.

Does the rise in uric acid during niacin therapy cause uric acid stones in the kidneys? No. Does it result in an increase in acute gouty arthritis? The Mayo group and I differed on this point; they believed niacin could precipitate episodes of acute gout and I didn't. The CDP didn't shed much light on this question. The average uric acid level in niacin participants was 6.75 at baseline and 6.80 at five years, really the same. The percentages of niacin patients having even one uric acid measurement outside certain limits during five years of study showed more men with uric acid levels above 8.0 or 10.0 than in those on placebo. Nothing new, since we already knew that niacin can elevate uric acid levels.

Did it matter clinically? The CDP report says, "The incidence of acute gouty arthritis was greater in the niacin group than in the placebo group." My good friend at the Mayo Clinic, Ken Berge, was on the CDP Writing Committee, so it is natural that his view would be reflected in the report; his experience and expertise with niacin exceeded that of all the other writers together. The report later says there was "no significant excess incidence of podagra, tophi, [or] uric acid stones in the niacin group." *Podagra* is the old medical term for acute gouty arthritis at the base of the great toe, the most common site for gout to strike. *Tophi* are small, hard nodules under the skin, composed of uric acid crystals, often on the rim of the ear cartilage but sometimes in or near joints. The fact that none of these evidences of gout occurred in so many men receiving niacin for at least five years supported my contention that there are few or no clinical consequences from niacin-induced hyperuricemia.

What, then, should a physician good at niacin do if uric acid levels are elevated during niacin therapy? *Stopping niacin is not necessary.* If the uric acid level exceeds 10.0, it is wise to reduce it with allopurinol, as it is in persons not receiving niacin. If a bout of acute gouty arthritis occurs, it should be treated with usual measures, nowadays a short course of a nonsteroidal anti-inflammatory agent (the group of which ibuprofen and naproxen are the most familiar to the public). It is not necessary to stop niacin in this situation either. There is no reason to avoid using niacin in a person with a history of gout or hyperuricemia.

Changes in Skin Other Than Flushing

Aside from cutaneous flushing early in treatment, especially with unmodified niacin, there are three side effects involving the skin. One of them occurs uniformly *(general dryness)*, one infrequently *(a nonspecific rash)*, and one rarely *(tan pigmentation of small areas)*.

Practically everyone who takes cholesterol-control doses of niacin for any length of time will have some degree of *dryness of the skin*. Although generalized, it will be more prominent in one area or another, often the trunk (back, abdomen) or lower calves. These areas tend to be dry anyhow, and niacin makes the tendency worse, especially in winter, when the sebaceous (oil) glands of the skin are less active.

Dermatologists tell me that the dryness occurs because the skin makes its own cholesterol, which is one of the skin's lubricants. Niacin inhibits cholesterol production wherever it occurs, including skin. I am not aware of any study which actually confirms this mechanism, but it really doesn't matter. This explanation makes sense, and the side effect is trivial.

Generalized skin dryness is seldom troublesome and should not deter treatment. Often the patient does not even notice that the skin is dry until I call attention to it during an examination. If dryness bothers the patient, the only treatment needed is a lubricating lotion. Any inexpensive hand or body lotion will work. It is not necessary to spend money on fancy dermatological products.

If a *skin rash* occurs, it can be more troublesome, depending on its characteristics. It can prevent ongoing use of niacin. As mentioned earlier, a slightly bumpy pink rash like mini-hives sometimes accompanies the cutaneous flush of niacin. This usually disappears early in treatment, as does the flush. However, some persons develop a pink, scaly rash which can be extensive, involving much of the body surface, particularly the trunk. Early in treatment, if flushing is still occurring, the rash may be accompanied by burning sensations, making some seek relief in a cold shower or bath or by

90

applying ice. More often, the rash will itch, and the skin may show scratch marks.

If this rash does not subside spontaneously, it will stop after discontinuing niacin. In a willing patient, a second trial may be worthwhile, but for many persons once is enough. Although one may decide to try a different preparation, TRNA instead of NA (or vice versa), the rash is likely to recur. The only recourse is to stop the drug permanently. I have not found oral antihistamines or local treatment of the rash with topical preparations to be worthwhile. So far I have not seen a rash caused by EP NA, after using the new product for about two years.

Tan pigmentation of local areas is a rare side effect of niacin. First reported in two of my Madison patients in 1959, these tan areas appeared along the periphery of the axillae (armpits) and along pressure areas such as the belt line and, in one man, where a winter jacket rubbed the sides of his neck. The involved skin areas appeared tan, slightly raised, with a velvety texture and appearance suggesting a skin disorder known as *acanthosis nigricans*. Others reported similar cases in other locations, including groins, antecubital and popliteal areas (the elbow fold and behind the knees). Biopsy results, reported in only a few cases, have been inconsistent, but some have reported microscopic changes compatible with acanthosis nigricans. In recent writings, it has become common to mention "acanthosis nigricans" as a side effect of niacin. Unless a biopsy has confirmed the microscopic appearance, I prefer to call it "a skin change *resembling* acanthosis nigricans."

These tan skin changes disappear following cessation of niacin therapy. However, discontinuation is not necessary unless the changes are cosmetically disturbing, which is seldom the case since they rarely appear on exposed surfaces.

Not all of niacin's effects on skin are undesirable. One very desirable effect was first demonstrated in two of my Madison patients and reported, with photographs, in 1959. Some persons with very high cholesterol levels develop hard deposits of cholesterol just under the skin or in tendons. These skin lesions, called *xanthoma tuberosum*, tend to occur on elbows and knees, sometimes on hands or buttocks. They are round nodules of various sizes, firm, often slightly yellow when the skin is stretched over them, only slightly movable, and sometimes confluent. *Xanthoma* means, literally, "yellow tumor." The two men I reported in 1959 had such deposits on their elbows and knees. In both men, the deposits softened in about a month and disappeared in about six months, never to return as long as they continued taking niacin.

One of these two men was the same one whose adventure with the insurance company concerning blood sugar levels we previously discussed. Figure 2 illustrated the overactivity of his body's cholesterol factory. He entered my study in 1956 at age 46. Soon thereafter, he had a heart attack; his cholesterol levels had not been controlled long enough to prevent it. After recovering uneventfully, he continued the niacin study.

When the CDP came along and our center joined it in 1967, he enrolled and happened to draw niacin as his CDP drug. By the time the CDP ended in 1974, I had moved to Scottsdale, so he continued taking niacin under the supervision of one of my former colleagues in Madison. He did not ever have a second heart attack. His leg arteries, already narrowed in 1956, did not ever disable him with any major blockage, allowing him to remain very active as a leader in the local curling club. He and his wife, both prominent in the community, served from time to time as hosts for foreign tours of the University of Wisconsin Alumni Association. In 1994, at age 83, he became ill with pneumonia and died in London, where they were leading an alumni tour.

His medical record taught us about reduction of cholesterol from very high levels, with elimination of skin xanthomas, and about the body factory's escape from control when niacin was stopped briefly or the correct dose reduced. More importantly, it showed the longevity and superb quality of life in a man who would probably have died prematurely without proper cholesterol control.

Another form of cholesterol deposit occurs in tendons: *xanthoma tendinosum*. Both this tendinous deposit and the skin xanthomas tend to occur in the most severe cases of hypercholesteremia, which are often familial (inherited). Even though their cholesterol levels are very high, persons with xanthomas are treated the same as any others, with follow-up of serum cholesterol levels and adjustment of the niacin dosage accordingly. Some of them also have elevated triglycerides *(mixed hyperlipidemia)*, but this doesn't matter because niacin reduces elevated triglycerides along with total and LDL cholesterol. As noted previously, no other lipid control drug has all of niacin's favorable properties.

In persons with xanthomas, reduction in serum cholesterol levels from very high values to normal levels occurs slowly. The levels do not reach normal within the first month or two, as in treatment of ordinary, moderate hypercholesteremia. Since reduction in cholesterol levels occurs during regression in the visible, palpable xanthomas, it seems reasonable to believe that the slower fall relates to removal of cholesterol from the xanthomas as well as reduction in current production by the body factory. The serum level would be lower sooner but for the resorption of the cholesterol deposits in skin. Since serum cholesterol usually does reach normal levels after months of proper dosage, a consistent downtrend in skin lesions and blood levels together should assure the physician that desirable changes are in progress and higher dosage is not needed.

Some people have a soft yellow plaque on an eyelid, called a *xanthelasma*. These are composed of cholesterol, and at one time it was thought that they indicated a high blood cholesterol level. Actually only about half of persons with xanthelasmata have hypercholesteremia, so the eyelid patch is not a reliable indicator. I have never paid much attention to whether such eyelid lesions disappeared with treatment or not, but I recall Dick Achor's telling me in the early days that they had seen complete disappearance of such lesions in one patient after two years of niacin therapy.

My 1959 report of reduction of xanthoma tuberosum in two patients was the first report of reduction in tissue cholesterol by niacin—or by any drug, since there were no others at the time. We expressed the hope that similar reduction might be occurring in arterial cholesterol-containing plaques but had no good way to measure them. We now know that such reduction does occur.

Visual Symptoms: Cystoid Macular Edema

There have been two reports (each with three patients) of a very infrequent side effect of niacin involving changes in vision. First reported by Donald Gass, M.D. (Miami) in 1973, the condition was characterized by swelling of the *macula*, the spot in the retina (back of the eye) which is the eye's center of sharpest vision. Symptoms were described as "like heat waves rising from hot pavement," or a sunburst or sunflower pattern in the middle of the visual field. The three men had trouble reading and following golf balls. They also noted fogginess and distortion of vision, brownish appearance of light bulbs, and patchy blind spots centrally. Symptoms began one month to one year after starting niacin. Examination showed an unusual swelling in the macula. As soon as Dr. Gass recognized this and stopped niacin, the visual changes rapidly recovered in one week to two months.

When discussing it with me, Dr. Gass called this rare disorder "the one cause of macular edema which always subsides when the relationship to a drug is recognized and the drug discontinued." He contrasted it to cystoid macular edema from chloraquine, a drug originally used to treat malaria, in which the disorder persists despite eliminating the causative agent.

The CDP performed annual eye examinations in all its patients for two to three years without finding any macular problems, so they stopped the expensive examinations. This experience was reassuring.

The other three cases of cystoid macular edema were reported in 1988 by eye doctors in Seattle and in Portland, Oregon, who found macular changes similar to those Gass had described. A fourth patient had visual symptoms but no retinal changes. In the eyes of 15 other patients taking niacin but with no symptoms, these physicians found no abnormalities. They correctly stated that patients taking niacin do not have to be screened for retinal problems unless they have symptoms. I agree, but I base my reasoning on CDP experience (1,100 men taking niacin), not on their 15 normal examinations.

Cystoid macular edema is a rare side effect of niacin. Anyone on cholesterol-control doses who experiences visual blurring or other ocular symptoms (central blind spots, sunburst or halos around lights) should be examined by an ophthalmologist. Because not every doctor, even eye specialists, may know about this problem, the knowledgeable patient should mention it if she has symptoms. The doctor might want to look up Don Gass's 1973 article in the *American Journal of Ophthalmology* (1973; 76: 500-510) or that of Millay and associates in *Ophthalmology* (1988; 95: 930-936).

Other Rare Side Effects

My detailed 1996 manuscript included a chapter titled *Side Effects and Other Problems Attributed to Niacin Infrequently or Incorrectly*. These are worth mentioning, just because they are rare and, if they ever should occur, might be missed by doctors who have not seen the articles I found. It is best, however, to include them in the Medical Section of this book. Interested readers can find them there; others will not be burdened by wading through them here.

Successful Management of Side Effects

How often should side effects, as discussed in this chapter, cause a patient or doctor to give up on use of niacin, the drug of first choice for cholesterol control? Not very often. Most patients will get over the flush early, or it will be prevented by use of aspirin and one of the modified niacin preparations (EP Plain Niacin or one of the leading TRNA preparations, Endur-acin or Slo-Niacin). Most will not be troubled by nausea. Queasiness or nausea will be managed skillfully by the physician. The doctor adept at using niacin will recognize that slight elevations of blood sugar, uric acid, or liver enzymes are unimportant parts of treatment.

Published studies by physicians good at niacin have had very low dropout rates, in the range of three to four per cent. This contrasts with the claim of niacin detractors, notably the representatives of companies selling other cholesterol-control drugs, that many people cannot take niacin successfully. In the CDP I taught principal investigators at the 53 centers, discussing niacin's use at the twice-yearly investigator meetings, supplemented with printed material. Some investigators cared enough to become good at niacin. Others cared less, so their participants had poorer adherence to full dosage of medication and more dropouts. Many centers, like the one I headed in Madison, had an excellent record of managing patients, owing to the combined effort of all the investigators. I have not kept score in 18 years of Madison studies and 20 years of Scottsdale practice, but the percentage of my patients who have successfully used niacin is probably greater that 90%.

In my opinion, doctors good at niacin will find that more than 90% of patients can use the drug comfortably and safely. This will bring these fortunate patients all the distinctive advantages of niacin and could reduce nationwide expenditures on drugs for cholesterol control by billions of dollars each year.

Summary

◆ Flushing of the skin from niacin can be minimized or eliminated entirely by preceding its use by a 325 mg aspirin tablet each morning and/or using time-release niacin (TRNA) or Endurance Products Plain Niacin (EP NA).

◆ If nausea occurs with niacin, adjusting the dose or the preparation used can allow many patients to receive the drug's benefits. Plain niacin causes less nausea than time-release products.

◆ Niacin does not cause or activate peptic ulcer.

◆ Minor changes in tests of liver function (enzyme levels less than twice the upper limit of normal) are a normal part of niacin therapy in some persons and do not require cessation of treatment.

◆ Elevations of liver enzyme values of two to three times the upper limit of normal require cessation of niacin therapy, which results in prompt return of the blood tests to normal.

◆ A patient with significant elevations of liver function tests on time-release niacin may be able to take plain niacin without similar problems.

◆ The minor elevations in blood glucose and uric acid which accompany use of niacin have no clinical significance and do not require its cessation or change in dosage.

◆ Niacin does not cause or "unmask" diabetes, but it should not be used in insulin-dependent diabetes.

◆ Previous history of peptic ulcer or of gout should not deter use of niacin.

◆ General dryness of skin always accompanies long-term niacin use and is easily managed by liberal application of lubricating lotions.

◆ A nonspecific skin rash from niacin may be troublesome enough to prevent its further use.

◆ A patient experiencing visual blurring, central blind spots, sunburst or halos around lights should be examined by an ophthalmologist (eye physician) because of the rare occurrence of cystoid macular edema, which subsides soon after niacin is discontinued.

◆ Doctors who have read this book and are thus good at niacin will be able to treat a high percentage of their hypercholesteremic patients (probably more than 90%) with niacin.

CHAPTER EIGHT

The Other Drugs for Cholesterol Control

To put current cholesterol-control drugs into perspective, one should remember that niacin was the first successful drug for this purpose, pioneered in 1955. As the years have gone by, its distinctive advantages have mounted. Each time the effects of various methods of treatment have been tested on newly discovered lipoproteins or subclasses, the results have turned out to be *more good news about niacin*. The drug has stood the test of time for more than 40 years. Not all drugs for lowering cholesterol have fared so well.

Triparanol (MER/29), marketed briefly in the late 1950's, was withdrawn from the market when it proved to cause cataracts. It also stopped synthesis (manufacture) of cholesterol at the last step before its immediate precursor, desmosterol, was converted to cholesterol. Desmosterol accumulated in the blood and was found in animals to be at least as dangerous as cholesterol in forming plaques in arteries.

The Coronary Drug Project stopped its use of *d-thyroxine (Choloxin)* because it caused more heart attacks than placebo. Although not ever used clinically, the commonly used female hormone *Premarin* was also included in the CDP in two dosage strengths, based on the observation that women had fewer heart attacks than men in those days, or at least had them later in life. The results showed that first the larger and then the smaller dose caused more clotting problems of all types, including heart attacks. Each dose was dropped from the study as soon as the results showed more hazard than placebo.

Although not removed from the market, *clofibrate (Atromid-S)* waned in popularity after the CDP. Even though it reached the finish line, along with niacin, its results showed no benefit in cardiovascular events, and it caused gallstones in some participants. Clofibrate is still used in Europe. Its relative, *gemfibrozil (Lopid)* is still marketed in the U.S. but has the same drawback (gallstones). We will discuss it briefly, along with the other current agents.

The most recent withdrawal has been *probucol (Lorelco)*, developed in the late 1960's and voluntarily removed from the U.S. market at the end of 1995. In 1993 the NCEP "Expert Panel" advised that use of probucol be restricted to patients who have not tolerated or not responded to other drugs. The Panel also said, "At present there is no clearly defined role for the use of probucol."

Besides niacin, there are only three groups of drugs for cholesterol control on the U.S. market now. Listed in order of their introduction (which matters, since a newly reported problem appeared in 1997 for one drug marketed in 1991), they are:

- Bile-sequestering resins (cholestyramine and colestipol)
- Fibrates (gemfibrozil)
- "Statins" (lovastatin, simvastatin, pravastatin, fluvastatin, and atorvastatin)

Bile-Sequestering Resins

In both the 1988 and 1993 NCEP guidelines, the "first-line drugs" recommended were niacin and the bile-sequestering resins. (In 1993 they changed the designation to "major drugs" and added the statins, of which three were then available.) The resins were usually mentioned first, since NIH in particular and other authors in general had always favored this order of preference, being niacin detractors at heart.

Two bile acid sequestrants are available, cholestyramine (Questran) and colestipol (Colestid). They are practically identical in action and efficacy.

To sequester means to remove or withdraw, to keep apart or isolate. The bile-sequestrant resins are granular (some would say sandy) particles which grab bile acids in the intestine, preventing them from being reabsorbed and recycled into cholesterol. Stirred into any liquid and ingested several times a day, they are capable of reducing LDLC and, therefore, total cholesterol. They do not raise HDLC or lower triglycerides, which may increase considerably, especially if the level is already elevated. The drugs are almost always intolerable to patients because they cause severe constipation, with accompanying bloating, flatulence, abdominal discomfort, and sometimes even nausea and vomiting.

Resins are not absorbed, a fact that appealed to their advocates, who reasoned that this meant that they could cause no harm. They just pick up bile acids on the surfaces of the granules and carry them out of the body. However, in similar fashion the resins interfere with absorption of various drugs (digoxin, anticoagulants, thyroxine, thiazide diuretics, beta blockers, and probably others). This makes it necessary to take other medications at least a couple hours away from the resin dose. Since the resin is taken several times a day, this is inconvenient, to say the least. If this precaution is not observed, resins may prevent absorption of very important medications, just listed.

In their 1988 guidelines, NCEP designated niacin and resins as "first-line drugs," based on their long safety records and their proven ability to reduce heart attacks. But had resins been clearly shown to reduce heart attacks and deaths? Let's look at the results of the large NIH-sponsored study on which such claims were based.

From 1973 to 1983 NIH conducted a study in 12 clinics throughout the U.S. called the Lipid Research Clinics Coronary Primary Prevention Trial, which I shall shorten to Lipid Research Clinic Trial (LRCT). In his book, George Mann called it "the most publicized and the most distorted trial…also the most expensive [$150 million] and, for several reasons, the most ominous of all the clinical trials…" I paraphrase here the summary he presented to support these statements. The reader must decide whether his judgment was too harsh.

The LRCT screened 480,000 men, aged 35 to 59 years, to find 3,806 suitable volunteers with cholesterol levels over 265. Mann points out that persons with cholesterol levels above 260 usually have an inherited disorder [familial hypercholesteremia], which occurs in only about one in forty American adults, so participants were not typical of the general population. The men were first given a low-fat, low-cholesterol diet for a short time, after which each was assigned to take either cholestyramine or a similar-appearing placebo powder. The groups were matched according to several risk factors in tests done before the study. The prescribed dose was six 4.0 g packets of powder each day, with adherence estimated by counting returned packets.

Dietary treatment alone lowered cholesterol levels by 4.6%, "a trivial effect." The added resin treatment lowered the levels by 13%. After 7.4 years of follow-up, the coronary heart disease (CHD) death rate was 30 (1.6%) in the treated group, 38 (2.0%) in the control group. By the statistical test specified in the protocol, this difference is not significant. (This means it could have occurred by chance in groups of this size.) Death from all causes was 68 (3.6%) in the resin group, 71 (3.7%) in the placebo group. This difference is far from significant. In four of the twelve clinics, no reduction of CHD events occurred, and in one clinic there were more CHD deaths in the resin group than in control subjects.

Mann goes on to say that when the study was begun in 1979, its "managers" proposed that levels of statistical significance be set at 0.01 because of the difficulty and cost of the study. [To the lay reader: Don't let this statistical gobbledygook throw you. Keep reading and you'll see the point.] In 1984, after they had seen the data, the managers raised the significance level to 0.05, which is easier to attain with a smaller difference between groups. Mann comments, "This is statistical cheating." Then, when reporting the findings, they changed again, using an entirely different statistical test! Mann again: "That is not acceptable practice. The operators adopted analytical methods to support their preconceived notion. This is not science but advocacy."

In 1992 the LRCT published a report of annual post-trial follow-up from 1985 to 1989 of about 1900 men each in resin and placebo groups. After just over 13 years of in-trial plus post-trial observation, there were 13 fewer deaths (143 vs.156) in the cholestyramine group. That difference is not statistically significant, which is nothing new for the LRCT. The authors concluded, "Overall, 6 years of post-[LRCT] follow-up have not provided conclusive evidence of benefit or long-term toxicity of cholestyramine treatment beyond that evident at the cessation of the trial."

From the LRCT came one of the silliest sayings about cholesterol ever to appear on the scene. Some one looked at the results and decided to say that "reducing cholesterol by 1% reduces the risk of heart attack by 2%." This became the catch-phrase for just about everyone to quote in support of cholesterol reduction, including the NCEP. I would be the last to say anything against cholesterol control, but to base it on LRCT findings, which had to undergo two changes in statistical methods to make the results look convincing, is ludicrous. The "1%-2% rule" is a Madison Avenue type of catch phrase to present its point glibly, but its basis is not sound.

Dwelling on the percentage change in total cholesterol and its fractions, which is common in the medical literature, does not make nearly as much sense as answering the question, *"Were the goals of treatment achieved?"* Percentages can be misleading since they are derived from baseline numbers of different sizes. Thus there will be greater percentage reduction in LDLC than in total cholesterol because the starting number is smaller. And when numbers are as small as HDLC levels are, especially when too low [below 35], seemingly large percentage changes may not be enough to achieve the goals of treatment, as already discussed. The 1%-2% rule may have served a purpose in calling attention to the importance of cholesterol measurement and control, but my reader knows by now that we should not accord it the reverence it has received.

Do the resins deserve to be recommended by the NCEP "Expert Panel" as a first-line drug, with the same stature as niacin? *I do not believe that they do.*

Resins are expensive. Cholestyramine (Questran) costs the patient about $86 a month (for three 4.0 g doses a day) to $172 per month for the LRCT target dose of 24 g per day. Likewise, colestipol (Colestid) costs $74 a month for three 5.0 g doses a day to $148 a month for six such doses per day.

Fibrates

Gemfibrozil (Lopid) is the only fibrate currently marketed in the U.S. As mentioned earlier, clofibrate may still be used in Europe, where one or more other fibrates are also available. Clofibrate, you recall, finished the CDP along with niacin but showed no cardiovascular benefits and caused gallstones in twice as many men as the placebo. A World Health Organization (WHO) study in Europe treated 5,000 subjects without known heart disease with clofibrate for five years and followed them for a sixth year. The clofibrate group had a significantly *higher* total mortality than a comparable placebo-treated group, due to a 33% increase in non-cardiovascular causes, including malignancy, post-cholecystectomy (gall bladder removal) complications, and pancreatitis.

Gemfibrozil has very limited indications (reasons to use the drug). Given as a 600 mg capsule twice daily, it was originally recommended by FDA only for the rare person with very high triglycerides (higher than 600 to 700 at least; some would say 900 to 1000, compared to a normal level of 200 or less). For some reason these very high levels present a risk for development of *pancreatitis*; lowering the circulating triglyceride level lessens this risk. Gemfibrozil is capable of reducing triglycerides and raising HDLC. It does not reduce LDLC levels.

A few years ago FDA required gemfibrozil's manufacturer to present FDA's recommendations by letter to every doctor in the U.S., apparently because FDA felt the drug was being promoted and used far beyond its clinical value. They advised that the drug be used only in patients with low

HDLC, high triglycerides, *and* high LDLC, and then *only if* the patient had not responded to diet, exercise, weight reduction, niacin, and bile sequestrants. (I am not sure why the resins were included in this list since they do not raise HDLC or reduce triglycerides.) FDA further stated that *if the goals are not attained* in two months, *the drug should be stopped.*

The only significant study of gemfibrozil has been a five-year trial in Finland, the Helsinki Heart Trial, sponsored by Warner Lambert, parent company of the drug's manufacturer, Parke Davis. Some would raise a question about the sponsorship, but who else is going to pay for it? A sponsor can affect the outcome of a study by carefully constructed protocols, excluding subjects unlikely to respond to the product or by analyzing data in a manner likely to show the product in the best light.

The Helsinki Heart Trial was a five-year randomized, double-blind study to compare the prevalence of coronary heart disease (CHD) and death in over 4,000 Finnish men with hypercholesteremia, treated with gemfibrozil or placebo. (A double-blind study is one in which neither the participant nor those running the trial know which subjects are receiving active drug and which placebo.) At entry all men were free of known CHD or symptoms and were 40 to 55 years of age.

All men had elevated cholesterol levels at entry. LDLC was above 175 in all, but triglycerides were normal in 63%. Both triglycerides and cholesterol were elevated in 28%; only triglycerides were elevated in the remaining 9%. Gemfibrozil reduced total cholesterol by only 11%, LDLC by only 10%, and triglycerides by 43%. HDLC increased by 10%. As a rule, these low levels of change are not clinically significant. More important would be whether the goals of treatment, by current NCEP guidelines, were achieved.

The rate of cardiac endpoints at five years was 4.1% in the placebo group and 2.7% in the gemfibrozil group, an overall reduction of 34%, which is significant. There was a lag period of about two years before the beneficial effect of medication emerged, just as the reduced death rate with niacin in the CDP only began to appear near the end of the study in men who had been followed for more than five years.

In spite of the differences in cardiac endpoints, *overall mortality rates did not differ.* The gemfibrozil group had more deaths from violence, accidents, and intracranial hemorrhage (bleeding within the head). This is one of the several diet or drug studies in which heart attack deaths were reduced but total deaths were equal in treated and placebo groups. The reason for this discrepancy is not known.

The Helsinki group published a later analysis (1992) which correlated various lipid measurements with the observed benefits. They found that the ratio of LDLC to HDLC was the best single predictor of cardiac events. This is worth remembering as we consider niacin, which changes both fractions in favorable directions.

In practice I sometimes use gemfibrozil (Lopid) if HDLC remains too low despite treatment with plain niacin (which increases HDLC more effectively than the time-release form, for some reason). I add the usual dose of gemfibrozil (600 mg twice a day) to the current niacin regimen. Even this combination may fail to bring HDLC to the desired level (higher than 45). In some cases, a value between 40 and 45 is the best we can do. If Lopid does not appear to contribute materially, it should be stopped after two months, as FDA specifies.

Lopid costs the patient about $73 a month. Generic gemfibrozil, available the last several years, costs about $30 a month. This makes this drug the least expensive agent except niacin, but its price is still about three times that of niacin, even for the generic form. More important to remember, as stated earlier, the drug has very limited usefulness.

HMG-Coenzyme A Reductase Inhibitors—The "Statins"

Lovastatin (Mevacor) was the first of a series of drugs which reduce cholesterol by inhibiting an enzyme (HMG-Coenzyme A reductase) which is needed for synthesis of cholesterol. The full name of the enzyme is "3-hydroxy-3-methyl-glutaryl-coenzyme A reductase," abbreviated as in the first sentence, or shortened to "co-A reductase." Here I will refer to its inhibitors as "statins," as doctors do in ordinary conversation, since each of their generic names ends in those two syllables.

At this writing, late in 1997, there are five statins on the market. Lovastatin (Mevacor), marketed in 1987, preceded the others by several years. Pravastatin (Pravachol) and simvastatin (Zocor) appeared in 1991. Fluvastatin (Lescol) came along in 1993.

Atorvastatin (Lipitor) was introduced early in 1997. In this discussion I shall call these agents by their brand names rather than the longer, easily confused, generic names.

These drugs have more similarities than differences. They have the same potential hazards. In fact, when *The Medical Letter*, an impartial publication which contains no advertising and reviews drugs knowledgeably, reviewed the second and third entries in this field, its experts warned practitioners that *if problems occur with one statin, there is no reason to believe that another can be used safely.* With further experience, this may change.

When Mevacor was first marketed, FDA required several warnings regarding its use. For a time, there was suspicion that the drug had caused cataracts in animals and in pre-marketing trials, so the FDA labeling called for yearly eye examinations. This requirement was removed late in 1991. The other warnings still apply.

Effects on Liver Function from Statins

The statins are capable of altering liver function tests with "marked, persistent increases in transaminase levels" (more than three times the upper limit of normal) in about 2% of patients receiving Mevacor for a year or more in early clinical trials. Later studies showed only 0.1% with "marked, persistent increases" on 20 mg or 40 mg per day and 1.5% at the maximum dose of 80 mg. The increases usually occurred after three to twelve months of treatment and were not associated with jaundice or other symptoms. After the drug was stopped, transaminase elevations *slowly* returned to normal, contrasted to *rapid* return if a similar situation occurs with niacin.

FDA formerly recommended that liver enzyme tests, including the SGPT (which is increased only by liver dysfunction, unlike some of the others) be done every six weeks for the first three months, every eight weeks through the rest of the first year, and at approximately six-month intervals thereafter. Later they relaxed the rules to six and twelve weeks after starting treatment, after each increase in dose, then "periodically"—which leaves further intervals to the physician's comfort level. FDA still advises caution in persons who drink much alcohol or have a history of liver disease.

George Mann's brief history of lovastatin's early development tells us, "In the 1960's the Japanese discovered a substance in a mold [actually a fungus—WBP] that inhibits the *in-vivo* synthesis of cholesterol from simple precursors. Since about 80% of body cholesterol comes from such precursors and not from diet, the notion was that the mold extract would block cholesterol synthesis and thus lower cholesteremia....But the Japanese found the substance (lovastatin) toxic in animal trials, and so they sold their process to Merck." I cannot vouch for the authenticity of this account, but it came from a scientist I know and trust.

Muscle Symptoms and Damage from Statins

A troublesome side effect of all statins, which is, fortunately, not very frequent, is a toxic effect on muscles, with several levels of severity. Its simplest form is *myalgia*, aching in muscles, not unlike the general aching, which often occurs with viral illness. When more severe, it becomes *myositis*, with actual inflammatory changes in muscles, accompanied by tenderness and rather marked elevations of CPK, an enzyme released from damaged muscle fibers. In its worst form, it becomes *rhabdomyolysis* (rab-doe-my-ALL-us-us), a destructive process in skeletal muscle fibers by dissolving the cell walls. The collective term for these several problems is *myopathy* (literally, "something wrong in muscles").

Fortunately, these muscle effects are relatively infrequent, with myositis reported in about 0.5% (1 in 200) of patients in clinical trials. Muscle problems are more likely to develop in patients also taking cyclosporine, a drug used to suppress rejection in heart transplant patients. Using statins in such patients is unwise because 50% develop the muscle complications. When gemfibrozil and lovastatin are used together, muscle problems occur in about 5%; with niacin and lovastatin together, about 2%. I know of no reason to expect different frequency with the other statins. The drugs are so competitive that we would have heard of any observed advantage.

In at least one reported case, the breakdown products from destruction of muscle fibers (rhabdomyolysis) caused kidney failure by blocking microscopic kidney tubules. The FDA warning says, "Consideration should be given to temporarily withholding or discontinuing drug therapy in any patient with a risk factor predisposing to the development of renal failure secondary to rhabdomyolysis, including: severe acute infection, hypotension [low blood pressure], major surgery, trauma, severe metabolic, endocrine, or electrolyte disorders and uncontrolled seizures." That's a scary sentence since it includes many situations, some of which are encountered fairly frequently.

The FDA labeling also reads, "Patients should be instructed to report promptly unexplained muscle pain or tenderness, particularly if accompanied by malaise and fever." Statin therapy should be stopped if markedly elevated CPK levels occur or myositis is diagnosed. It does not help to measure CPK levels in patients taking statins unless muscle symptoms occur. *Enzyme levels cannot be used to predict myopathy* or to reassure the physician that it is not going to occur.

Two things bother me about the statins, one regarding myopathy and CPK changes, the other regarding drug interactions which greatly increase the muscle effects. Not many of my patients take statins. Probably 90% or more of my patients take niacin for their cholesterol problems. In those who do not tolerate niacin, statins are my choice for those with too much LDLC and TC, the most common cholesterol abnormality. In my relatively few patients taking these drugs, I have seen *four* persons develop myopathy. Each had myalgia, sometimes with tenderness and one patient with weakness as well. *None of the four had an elevated serum CPK level*, and yet I am certain clinically (including slow reversal of symptoms after stopping the drug) that each had statin myopathy. Hold that thought in mind. We'll come back to it.

In protocols for studies of statins, it is customary to measure serum CPK levels and to brand a situation "myopathy" *only if these levels exceed ten times normal*. If that criterion, rather than the occurrence of clinical symptoms, is used to count the cases of myopathy, the incidence of muscle problems will be grossly understated, judging from my clinical experience. This may be one example of a way in which drug companies sponsoring studies can influence the ground rules and minimize reporting of adverse findings. None of my four patients with myopathy would have been counted!

In 1994 Merck mounted an aggressive advertising campaign which included full-page newspaper ads in many markets across the country. (More about these expensive campaigns later.) One of my patients, a middle-aged woman who had failed to tolerate niacin and had received Mevacor for a while, mailed me one of the full-page newspaper ads. At the bottom she had printed, "The medicine that gave me the myopathy. No fun to feel helpless. Just getting over another siege." I had not known until then that the muscle symptoms could recur even without further use of the statin.

A New, Frightening Problem

What is my other recent concern about the statins? Mevacor has been on the market only since 1987, Pravachol and Zocor only since 1991, Lescol only since 1993, and Lipitor only since early 1997. New adverse effects are still being uncovered. In the first quarter of 1997, a letter to the editor of *JAMA (Journal of the American Medical Association)* reported a newly observed problem, a drug interaction that can greatly increase the effects of statins, sometimes with drastic results.

A 44-year-old man was taking simvastatin (Zocor), 40 mg a day, under the care of lipidologists (cholesterol specialists) at the University of Cincinnati, who customarily saw him at three-month intervals. His family physician, supervising the remainder of his care, prescribed a new antidepressant, nefazodone (Serzone). One month later the patient returned to his doctor, complaining of passing tea-colored urine. Not recognizing a potentially serious problem, the doctor thought he had a urinary infection and treated him with an antibiotic. When the patient returned to the Lipid Clinic after another month, he still had brown urine, plus severe myalgias in his thighs and calves. Dr. Charles Glueck (a well-known cholesterol researcher for many years) and his associates recognized that the tea-colored urine was caused by excretion of myoglobin, a product of muscle breakdown (rhabdomyolysis), resulting from the statin. Test results, including very high serum levels of myoglobin and muscle enzyme CPK, verified this diagnosis.

But there's more to this situation than just the infrequent myopathy from statins. Numerous drugs, including statins, are metabolized (removed from circulation and broken down) by liver enzymes known as the P450 group. Quite a number of commonly used drugs can *inhibit* the P450 enzymes, preventing them from handling not only statins but also a considerable list of other drugs. Among the P450 inhibitors are Serzone and its older, better-known relatives: Prozac, Zoloft, and Paxil. By prescribing Serzone in a patient receiving Zocor, the family physician unwittingly caused a huge build-up of the statin drug. This caused destruction of muscle, with sky-high CPK levels, and myoglobin in the urine.

Statins are the most frequently prescribed agents for hypercholesteremia. The group of antidepressants of which Prozac was the first and Serzone is the latest is the most effective for depression. What other drugs inhibit P450 enzymes and could result in the same effect—that of a great overdose of the statin? On the list are macrolide antibiotics, including erythromycin and its newer, more powerful cousin, Biaxin. These are good choices for common respiratory infections, ranging from sinusitis to bronchitis and pneumonia. Agents used for fungal infections, such as ketoconazole and fluconazole, are on the list. So are calcium channel blockers verapamil and diltiazem, frequently used for high blood pressure or heart problems, which often coexist with hypercholesteremia. Even *grapefruit juice* is an inhibitor of one P450 enzyme and could cause trouble in an unfortunate patient drinking it while taking a statin!

The recent discovery of such a serious adverse effect in a drug on the market for only six years (Zocor), in a group of drugs whose oldest member has been available for only ten years, underlines the importance of niacin's safety record of more than four decades. It also makes one realize that other adverse reactions to statins might yet appear.

Do Statins Adversely Affect Mental Performance?

Remember the Helsinki Heart Trial's report that, although cardio-vascular events were reduced, the total death rate was the same with gemfibrozil as with placebo, due in part to increases in deaths from violence and accidents? Cholesterol reduction has also been associated with increased deaths from accidents, violence, and suicide in other studies, leading some to believe that reducing cholesterol too much might be responsible. (See The Medical Section, *Are Low Cholesterol Levels Harmful?* for further discussion.)

At the November 1997 American Heart Association meeting, Muldoon and his associates at my alma mater, University of Pittsburgh, reported a study comparing the effects of lovastatin and placebo on various aspects of mental function in hypercholesteremic patients. They used the usual starting dose of lovastatin, 20 mg daily, for six months and achieved the expected reduction in TC (18%) and LDLC (23%).

Cognitive performance on tests of mental flexibility, working memory, and memory recall were unaffected, but lovastatin treatment caused decreases in attention and psychomotor speed, compared to placebo. Subjects with the greatest cholesterol reduction also showed the greatest declines in cognitive performance. They concluded that reduction in serum cholesterol might have adverse effects on tasks requiring sustained attention and psychomotor speed, but whether such treatment effects alter performance on tasks of everyday life, such as automobile driving, remains to be seen. Clearly, more study is needed. But this report is another example of a possible new adverse effect of a drug in widespread use but only on the market for ten years.

Effects of Statins on Serum Lipids

All statins reduce total cholesterol and LDLC. Although FDA apparently allows manufacturers to say that the drugs raise HDLC, the increases are too small (8% to 15%) to be clinically significant. If below 35, low HDLC is an independent risk factor for coronary disease. (This means that even if everything else is fine, a person with HDLC this low is at considerable risk.) With treatment, we can't just achieve a level of 36 and heave a sigh of relief; we should bring the HDLC level to 45 or higher. Suppose the HDLC level without treatment is 30. To raise it 8% to 15% means an increase of only 2.4 to 4.5; this leaves the HDLC fraction below 35, still in a dangerous range. That's what I mean by "not clinically significant."

Early Regression Studies with Mevacor

Mevacor has not been shown to reduce coronary heart disease endpoints or death in a large prospective trial like the CDP, which demonstrated niacin's success in these matters. However, there have been new methods of demonstrating changes in arteries, including measurement of cholesterol plaques to detect progression or regression. Most studies of arterial diameter have compared coronary arteriograms before and after two years or more of treatment.

A Los Angeles group led by the late David Blankenhorn performed two of the most impressive regression studies. Their Cholesterol Lowering Atherosclerosis Study (CLAS) was the first of about ten studies to show that various interventions for cholesterol control could lessen existing coronary artery plaques (regression) in addition to retarding new deposits. Using niacin and colestipol resin (the "first-line" drugs of the 1988 NCEP guidelines), the researchers showed that the drug combination had a beneficial effect on coronary artery cholesterol deposits after two years and after four years.

In their second study, Monitored Atherosclerosis Regression Study (MARS), Blankenhorn and associates used the maximum dose of Mevacor, 80 mg per day. Average arterial narrowing increased slightly in those on placebo but decreased 4.1% in those taking this large Mevacor dose. The scoring system, based on expert reading of the arteriograms, showed regression in 13 placebo recipients and in 28 patients taking Mevacor. The amount of regression was slight, but remember that flow experts say it doesn't take much increase in diameter to produce a significant increase in flow of blood.

Another study, expensive and oft-quoted by Merck in its advertising, was the Expanded Clinical Evaluation of Lovastatin (EXCEL), reported in 1990 and 1991. In 362 sites in U.S. (an unwieldy situation), investigators followed more than 8,000 persons in five groups of 1,600 or more. The groups received either placebo or Mevacor in doses from 20 mg to 80 mg a day. When more than 20 mg was given, the results were better if the drug was given in divided doses rather than all at once in the evening. Reductions in total and LDL cholesterol were dose-related. HDLC did not increase significantly. The protocol excluded persons with elevated triglycerides or low HDLC, which often go together and do not respond well to lovastatin. Studies like this one, performed at an unwieldy number of locations, allows the sponsoring company to receive and control all the data, from which it can extract whatever favorable results it chooses.

Mevacor costs the patient about $65 a month for the usual starting dose of 20 mg a day and as much as $210 a month if the maximum dose of 80 mg is required. Merck's patent on the drug expires in 1999, and no one knows how this will affect the statin market. The company, which has another entry in the field (simvastatin, or Zocor), has not been promoting Mevacor very actively in the past few years, preferring to concentrate on its younger product, which has longer patent protection. For a long time I used Mevacor, on the market longer, in preference to the more recently introduced products since their results were comparable. (Of course, most of my patients take niacin, so relatively few use statins.) In the past couple years my tendency has been to use whichever statin(s) the patient's HMO formulary or pharmacy plan covers.

The Next Two Statins: Pravachol and Zocor

Mevacor had the statin field to itself from 1987 to 1991, in which year two more drugs entered the marketplace. Bristol-Myers Squibb marketed Pravachol (pravastatin) the same year that Merck marketed Zocor (simvastatin).

When first studied, both drugs were found to have several side effects which are usually mild and transient but deserve mention. These include headache, gastrointestinal cramps, constipation, nausea, and flatulence. Pravachol also caused occasional skin rashes. A German group reported "inflammatory myopathy" from pravastatin; it appears that all the statins have this potential side effect, which could be intensified by interaction with certain other drugs, as discussed earlier (Glueck's patient in Cincinnati who received Zocor with an antidepressant). An Austrian group cited four cases of depression in women receiving pravastatin, prompting a rebuttal letter from the manufacturer, saying that 14 studies around the world (2,485 patients) did not support such an association.

Both Pravachol and Zocor have been studied in combination with cholestyramine resin. In both instances the combination showed an increased effect. The reports emphasized that the statin must be taken at least an hour away from each resin dose, so the resin will not pick up the other drug and interfere with its absorption. Obviously the statins should be added to the list of important drugs on which the resins have this effect.

The results of the Scandinavian Simvastatin Survival Study, reported at the November 1994 American Heart Association meeting, have been among the most impressive to date. Sponsored by Merck, Zocor's manufacturer, the study was performed in 94 centers in Sweden, Norway, Denmark, Finland, and Iceland. I still suspect that such a widespread study would be unwieldy to manage, compared to the tight control of the CDP, in which I played a part. The positive results and the catchy short designation ("4S Study") captivated the press and the medical world. Over a five-year period, the investigators followed 4,444 (another catchy feature) men and women, 35 to 70 years of age. Each already had coronary disease, as evidenced by anginal pain or previous heart attack. After a preliminary diet phase, cholesterol levels were between 212 and 309. [Keep noticing that preliminary diet, sometimes shortened to "run-in diet" in investigator jargon, never does much. Investigators include it in their protocols to be politically correct because diet advocates still wield influence. Some would say to fail the "try diet first" test might impair receiving a research grant or having a paper accepted for publication. Observing the NCEP "start with diet" advice protects the authors from possible criticism, or even rejection, from a journal whose editorial reviewers might be offended if diet were not given its due. This preliminary phase lets investigators say, in effect, "We tried it and it didn't work; now let's get on with our study." It also avoids criticism that part of any achieved success was due to dietary change, not drug effect.]

Persons with elevated triglycerides were excluded. As mentioned previously, this provision tends to exclude persons with low HDLC, which statins do not help. This tends to improve the resulting data. The starting dose of 20 mg Zocor was increased to 40 mg in 37% of those taking the drug. Zocor decreased total and LDL cholesterol but did not raise HDLC significantly, as usual. During five years, 256 patients in the placebo group died, compared to 182 in the Zocor group. Coronary disease caused death in 189 placebo patients, 111 on Zocor. The drug was well tolerated, with few dropouts. There was no increase in non-cardiovascular deaths in the drug group, so it cannot be incriminated in causing mysterious accidental deaths and suicides, as in some diet and drug studies.

The pre-arranged press coverage of the report at the AHA meeting resulted in a media blitz of favorable publicity for simvastatin (Zocor). When the incoming AHA president praised the study as the first to show that drug therapy of hypercholesteremia could actually reduce deaths and cardiovascular events, she chose to overlook the CDP results, which clearly showed such benefits from niacin. The Oslo coordinator of the 4S study was quoted as saying that the study was the first to demonstrate beyond doubt that physicians can use "a well-tolerated medicine" to alter the course of coronary disease and help patients with coronary disease live longer. If reported accurately, this dig at niacin and resins is unbecoming.

In a promotional cassette tape sent to doctors by Merck, those discussing the 4S Study boasted that the drug cost per patient was *only $6,000* for five years of study. They considered this cost quite reasonable when compared to the high costs of a heart attack, coronary bypass surgery, angioplasty, or other procedures. At $10 per month, the cost of niacin for five years would be $600, *exactly one-tenth* of the estimated cost for simvastatin! And no matter what the reported success of the statins, they do not do the distinctive things niacin does by raising HDLC (especially HDL$_2$), favorably altering particle sizes in subfractions of LDLC, and reducing Lp(a).

The manufacturers of Pravachol and of Zocor have been very active in sponsoring expensive studies, seeking to gain FDA approval for impressive advertising claims which might give them larger shares of the multi-billion dollar cholesterol-control market. In fact, there has been a traffic jam of acronyms, with two studies of Pravachol abbreviated "PLAC," forcing them to be called PLAC-1 and PLAC-2. At the 1994 AHA meeting (always in November), Dr. Bertram Pitt's Ann Arbor group reported PLAC-1 (Pravastatin Limitation of Atherosclerosis in the Coronary Arteries), "the first study of a [statin] to demonstrate convincingly both regression of atherosclerotic lesions as detected by angiography and the reduction of coronary events." (Recall my saying that Mevacor had not been shown to reduce cardiovascular events.)

In PLAC-2 (Pravastatin, Lipids, and Atherosclerosis in the Carotids), Byington and associates (Winston-Salem) measured carotid neck arteries by ultrasound in 151 patients with previous heart attack or at least 50% narrowing in a coronary artery. Although those who took Pravachol (10 to 40 mg per day) showed LDLC reduction (166 to 120), there was gradual *progression* of average carotid artery thickness by ultrasound. Progression, measured in 12 selected segments of carotid artery wall, was *not* significantly slower with pravastatin, but the rate of progression in the *common* carotid artery (the large artery low in the neck, before it branches) was 54% less. During three years of study, ten of 76 in the placebo group had heart attacks, compared to four of 75 on Pravachol.

A group at University of Kuopio in Finland performed another early study (1989-1992), and investigators from Leiden, Netherlands reported in 1994 and 1995 a study which included more patients (884) than PLAC-1 and PLAC-2 combined. The Leiden trial had, of course, a catchy acronym,

REGRESS (Regression Growth Evaluation Statin Study). In general, these trials showed the same findings as all the rest.

As with the 4S Study in 1994, AHA again spotlighted a glamour study at its 1995 meeting, with the same exorbitant media coverage and pre-arranged publication in a leading medical journal. This time it was the West of Scotland Coronary Prevention Study, which compared Pravachol and placebo in 6,600 middle-aged men who had not had a heart attack, although 10% had angina (heart-related chest pain) and 6% had exertional leg pains from poor circulation. The Pravachol dose was set at 40 mg a day to assure good results, rather than titrating it according to cholesterol response. Average LDLC fell from 192 to 142 with the drug. As in most studies, the report did not say how many men reached the goals of treatment. During almost five years of follow-up, there were 248 coronary events (nonfatal heart attacks or death from CHD) in the placebo group but only 174 in the Pravachol group. There were no excessive deaths from non-cardiovascular causes. Risk reduction extended to patients without multiple risk factors and those without preexisting vascular disease.

We have already noted the Madison Avenue aspects of the 4S Study, part of its multi-million dollar promotion after the 1994 AHA meeting. Now the 1995 meeting spotlighted the West of Scotland Study. Speakers love to say its name, which rolls off the tongue like the fog across the moors. I have wondered if it would have achieved such popularity if called by its eponymic abbreviation, WOSCOPS. Most important for Bristol-Myers Squibb, it won FDA approval for the claim that Pravachol was capable of preventing first heart attacks. Since then the company has touted this claim with ads costing millions of dollars, aimed at the public as well as doctors.

Of course, Merck has also been very active in the race for market shares with Zocor ads, many of them aimed at the public. Notable has been their series of TV spots which roll a list of unappealing slang terms they have coined for cholesterol: blood mud, artery goo, coronary sludge, and the like. I called the 800 number and received a series of three mailings in the following two weeks, each including at least one color brochure on hard paper, giving general information about cholesterol and telling the patient, "Give your doctor this cholesterol test." It then advises anyone with "high cholesterol," being treated with diet and exercise, to ask the doctor six questions: Has my treatment program of diet and exercise sufficiently reduced my high cholesterol? If not, is it appropriate for me to add a cholesterol-lowering medication to my diet and exercise plan? What medication (if any) is appropriate for me? How long should I take it? What are the side effects? What kinds of results can I expect?

On their list of risk factors for heart disease, they lead off with high LDL cholesterol, followed by smoking, high blood pressure (treated or untreated), diabetes, age (man over 45, woman over 55), family history, and (at the end of the list) low HDL cholesterol. Low HDLC is never mentioned again. You know the reason: statins do not improve this situation.

Zocor TV ads have portrayed a middle-aged man helping his grandchild on a bicycle—unless, of course, he has a young wife and this is his child. The same photo has been used in magazine advertising, sometimes with the admonition, "Be there!" Their ads are based on the 4S Study. Meanwhile, Pravachol ads have emphasized its ability to lessen the likelihood of first heart attacks. Does this mean that niacin or the other statins do not have the ability to prevent first heart attacks or to prolong the life of that gray-haired gentleman? *Of course not!* It is very likely that *all* statins have the properties demonstrated for any one of them in these expensive studies, *and so does niacin.*

FDA grants a claim to the company which submits evidence of what its drug can accomplish—for example, prevent first heart attacks (Pravachol), or reduce heart attacks and deaths (Zocor). Niacin was shown in the CDP to reduce heart attacks, strokes, cardiovascular surgery, and total deaths in men with one or more previous heart attacks (secondary prevention). Does this mean that the drug is not effective in primary prevention? On the contrary, it probably is effective, but such a study has not been done for nonpatentable niacin, which is not making any company rich. If one were to speculate, niacin, because of its distinctive advantages, probably does a better job of preventing events than the statins.

The proliferation of expensive studies and competition for market shares really does the patient no favors. It just increases the prices of the expensive drugs, notably the statins. Obviously studies as large as the 4S Study and WOSCOPS are extremely expensive. Who do you think paid for those studies and for the outlandish expenditures on TV and print advertising? If you said Merck and Bristol-Myers Squibb, you are wrong. *All these bills were paid by patients who have spent money on their products to date and will do so in the future. Do not look for the prices of these statins to come down very soon.*

One more Pravachol study, reported at a meeting early in 1996 and reviewed at the AHA meeting that November, was called Cholesterol and

Recurrent Events, or CARE. [Don't you love these acronyms?] This five-year multicenter study in U.S. and Canada enrolled more than 4,000 men and women with recent heart attacks and total cholesterol levels less than 240 (average 209). In addition to the drugs for cholesterol control, they continued to receive other desirable post-heart attack treatment. Participants were randomized to Pravachol 40 mg (the maximum recommended dose) or placebo for a five-year study. Pravastatin reduced heart attack or death from coronary disease and the need for coronary bypass or balloon angioplasty, each by about 25%. The study's chairman Braunwald (Boston), said that this trial was the first to focus on persons with cholesterol levels less than 240, which is important since 75% of heart attack survivors have TC levels in this range. If he had recalled the CDP, he would have realized that more than half of its participants, all heart attack survivors, had TC levels less than 250 at baseline. Then he might also have had to remember that niacin reduced both heart attack and stroke by about 25% and cardiovascular surgery by 46%, not a bad record for an old, established drug given in a less than optimal dose.

The study's leaders calculated that for every 1,000 patients treated for five years in CARE, 153 cardiac events were avoided. In women, 248 events were avoided for each 1,000 treated. They tended to gloss over the fact that 12 women taking pravastatin developed breast cancer during the study, compared with only one woman in the placebo group. "Probably a statistical fluke," they said, given the fact that such a problem was not seen in previous large trials of pravastatin or related drugs. However, the huge difference, twelve to one, is quite a large fluke, if that's what it is. The breast cancer matter deserves close observation in future use of all the statins.

Later Arriving Statins: Lescol and Lipitor

Lescol (fluvastatin), marketed by Sandoz in 1993, was the first completely synthetic statin, which means that the others must be produced, at least in part, by the "mold" [fungus] George Mann mentioned. At first it seemed that Lescol worked about as well as the other statins and sold at a lower price. More recently it appears that you may get what you pay for, that Lescol is not as capable as the other statins of reducing TC and LDLC in persons with difficult cholesterol factories. Some are now advising that Lescol be used in persons with relatively mild hypercholesteremia and the other, more effective statins in those with more severe problems.

Managed care groups like so-called "Health Maintenance Organizations" often have Lescol on their formularies to the exclusion of its more expensive relatives. Even though Lescol's $44 monthly cost seems low in comparison to other statins, let's not forget that niacin costs much less, at $8 to $10 a month, and offers advantages the statins do not have.

Lipitor was introduced by Parke-Davis in January 1997, having been heralded at the November AHA meeting as a different statin. Besides the usual actions on TC and LDLC, it also reduces triglycerides, but its meager elevation of HDLC (5% to 9%) is as unimpressive as the action of the other statins on this fraction. In clinical studies at the starting dose of 10 mg a day, Lipitor achieved somewhat better reductions in TC, LDLC, and triglycerides than any of the other statins. Of course, the impact on clinical outcomes (heart attacks, strokes, other atherosclerotic events) of these small differences is not known and may not be very great.

The starting dose of 10 mg daily costs $55 a month. Higher doses (20 mg, 40 mg, 80 mg) cost from $83 to $222 a month. Like all statins, it is not recommended in severe liver disease or persons using much alcohol. Liver function studies need to be monitored. The doctor needs to warn his patient of possible myopathy. FDA issues the same scary warning list of factors which might predispose to chronic kidney failure as discussed for the other statins. In pre-clinical trials, the drug was generally well tolerated, with adverse reactions including constipation, flatulence, indigestion, and abdominal pain. We have to assume that inhibitors of the P450 enzymes might cause a tremendous build-up of the drug, as in Glueck's patient on Zocor and Serzone. The doctor must be alert to this possibility for all statins.

Lipitor may turn out to be the best of the statins, but its limited post-marketing experience means that it could have unpredicted adverse effects not seen with related drugs which have been on the market four, six, or ten years longer than it has. Time will tell.

At present the statins are the best choice for patients who do not tolerate niacin, and there will be some, even in the hands of doctors good at niacin. Use of statins should be limited to persons who need reduction in TC and LDLC since these drugs offer no benefit in those with low HDLC levels. Which statin to choose? Mevacor has the longest safety record and may become generic in 1999. How this will affect pricing is anybody's guess. The fact that Pravachol can boast, with FDA's blessing, of preventing first heart attacks (or reducing their incidence, to be more exact) does not mean that this is the only statin or the only cholesterol-control drug with this characteristic. Probably all the statins and niacin can do the same thing. Zocor's lessening of heart attacks and deaths in the 4S Study is not an exclusive property, either. We have already observed that niacin did about as well in the CDP at suboptimal doses, and the other statins probably could perform as well.

Lipitor is the only statin which shares niacin's ability to reduce triglycerides along with LDLC and TC, but it is not clear that such reduction lessens cardiovascular events, and it will never really be known. Triglycerides are unimportant as a risk factor for atherosclerotic disease and may be just a marker for diabetes (which develops later in many people with high triglycerides). A few experts think triglycerides combine with obesity in women to present an increased risk of coronary disease, but both conditions respond to weight reduction, so we need not be overly concerned.

Whether Lipitor proves to be slightly more effective, dose for dose, than the other statins remains to be seen. And if it is, whether that means fewer events is also unknown.

Like its predecessors, Lipitor was introduced with a huge splash. Eight-page ads in medical journals started in January and were still running in May. Like all its competitors, this drug's manufacturer, Parke-Davis, spared no expense, spending millions to grab a share of the billions which people in U.S. spend on statins each year. We know who pays and how this affects drug prices, don't we?

I don't know the current cost of a page of advertising in leading medical journals, but it is plenty. Years ago (in the early 1960's) I was talking with officers of a company that manufactured a niacin product we had been testing. I had been annoyed by the amount of junk mail we constantly received and was complaining about it. The company's vice-president explained to me the reason for so much direct advertising, saying, "I can send a mailing to every doctor in the country six times for what it costs me to run a one-page ad in the *JAMA*."

The explanation has always stuck with me, giving a general idea of the amounts drug companies spend on print advertising. When the companies take their messages to the public with TV ads, the cost is even greater.

Estrogens

Using estrogen replacement therapy in postmenopausal women to help prevent osteoporosis has been associated with a favorable effect on coronary disease and cardiovascular death in most observational studies. But these have not been randomized controlled studies; groups were not matched beforehand, and the benefits are open to question. To be effective in osteoporosis, the daily estrogen dose must be at least 0.625 mg of conjugated equine estrogens (Premarin) or its equivalent. One new study (December 1997) says that half this dose may be successful. Women taking more than 1.25 mg per day show less benefit and possibly some adverse effects, consistent with the CDP's adverse findings in men with previous heart attacks who took 1.25 or 2.5 mg.

Estrogens increase HDLC levels, but this probably explains only a small part of their beneficial effect. In an earlier chapter we noted that estrogens reduce Lp(a) in postmenopausal women, the only agent besides niacin to alter this risk factor.

Estrogen should not be used to treat any lipid disorder but might be considered if a postmenopausal woman not taking estrogen has low HDLC which does not respond to niacin. The main question, as with use of estrogens to reduce osteoporosis, is the risk of cancer. If a woman still has her uterus, adding progesterone to estrogen reduces the risk of uterine cancer to an acceptable level but does not eliminate it. Estrogens do increase the risk of breast cancer, and many women prefer to take their chances with osteoporosis rather than incur this added risk. I do not blame them and do not push the use of hormones. Breast tenderness and fluid retention, which can cause abdominal bloating and ankle swelling, make estrogens intolerable for some women.

For my postmenopausal women, I outline the broad picture of lessening osteoporosis (which we can't prevent!). Each woman should really have started in adolescence, making sure that the daily intake of calcium was adequate (1000 mg daily before menopause and 1500 mg after) and that regular weight-bearing exercise was adequate, daily or nearly so. Other risk factors include petite stature, heavy smoking, or alcohol use; the first is not under our control. In my view, estrogen replacement is not utterly essential if a woman does not want it or does not tolerate it well. Regular weight-bearing exercise and adequate calcium intake are important and are available to every woman.

Summary

◆ Bile acid sequestrants (cholestyramine and colestipol) are capable of reducing total cholesterol and LDLC but do not change HDLC or triglycerides. If the inconvenience of stirring these sandy products into liquids and drinking the suspension several times a day does not drive the patient away, uncomfortable gastrointestinal symptoms usually do. In addition, resins must be taken at least an hour apart from other important medicines to be sure they do not interfere with absorption. Resins are expensive.

118

◆ The LRC trial did not demonstrate a statistically significant reduction in nonfatal heart attacks and deaths in those receiving cholestyramine, but two changes in the statistical methods produced figures more to the liking of NHLBI, determined to have a success story to tell at the press conference. George Mann calls this "statistical cheating." I say that resins have too many things going against them to be designated a "first-line drug."

◆ Gemfibrozil can reduce triglycerides and may increase HDLC but seldom normalizes the lipid profile. It does not reduce TC or LDLC; in fact, it has been reported to increase LDLC. FDA has tried to tell doctors that this drug is overpromoted and overused. There is little or no justification for using gemfibrozil in clinical practice.

◆ Lovastatin (Mevacor) can reduce TC and LDLC. It does not cause clinically significant increases in HDLC, reduce Lp(a), or favorably alter the LDL subfractions. It has lessened progression and produced some degree of regression in coronary plaques. Although no study has shown that it can lessen heart attacks and deaths, it probably shares this property with other statins. Its safety record, more than ten years, exceeds that of the other statins. Its use requires laboratory monitoring for liver toxicity and clinical monitoring for myopathy, which cannot be predicted by CPK determinations. This drug is a reasonable choice for patients who, for one reason or another, cannot take niacin, but its limitation in treating low HDLC should be remembered. Mevacor is expensive. Merck's patent on lovastatin will expire in 1999.

◆ The other statins—Pravachol (pravastatin), Zocor (simvastatin), Lescol (fluvastatin), and newcomer Lipitor (atorvastatin)—share Mevacor's strengths and weaknesses. Lipitor differs by being the only statin which reduces triglycerides, for whatever value that may have. Each of the drugs except Lipitor has caused regression in arterial plaques and some (Zocor, Pravachol) have reduced heart attacks and deaths. It is likely that all statins, as well as niacin, have all of these favorable effects.

◆ All statins require the same monitoring for liver toxicity and myopathy as does lovastatin. Workers in this field are still trying to sort out the significance of several infrequent side effects. If a patient has trouble with one statin, there is no evidence that it is safe to use another.

◆ Even Lescol, the least expensive statin, is several times higher in price than niacin.

◆ Estrogens, when used for menopausal symptoms or to lessen osteoporosis, may help the lipid profile by increasing HDLC. There have been no prospective studies involving cardiovascular endpoints, but there is a general belief that fewer heart attacks have occurred in observational studies of women taking estrogens.

◆ None of the other drugs reduces Lp(a) or alters HDLC subfractions or LDLC subfractions favorably, as niacin does.

CHAPTER NINE

What Can I Say to My Doctor to Be Sure He Is Good at Niacin?

You now understand why niacin is far preferable to the other drugs for treating cholesterol problems. You know what you need to find out about your lipid profile to decide whether you need treatment. But you also know that niacin is not a do-it-yourself drug. It requires knowledgeable medical supervision.

If your doctor has not measured your bad and good cholesterol fractions and treated them to target levels, what can you say to him? What can you say if he says he is afraid to use niacin because it causes terrible flushing or liver damage? Or if he has you taking one of the other drugs, which may or may not be achieving the goals of treatment—the resins, with their major defects, or a statin, which does not have niacin's distinctive advantages in regard to newly discovered lipid fractions? Or if you are spending large amounts of money each month on other drugs when niacin could do everything right—inexpensively and without diet? How can you present your desire to take niacin and at the same time be sure he is good at using the drug?

As I said at the outset, you need to buy another copy of this book and give it to your doctor. (You will want to keep yours to refer to and show your friends.) Don't worry that he may have received a copy from some one else. He will value it because it came from you, and he may choose to use an extra copy to present the information to another patient. If the book comes from only one patient, he may put it aside and not read it. But if several patients give him the book with glowing recommendations, he may decide he should take it seriously and at least read it. You may play a part in bringing the benefits of niacin to others, as well as yourself.

Before considering what to say, it is well to decide what you plan to do if your doctor rejects your suggestion out of hand and shoves the book back across the desk to you. Some doctors are prima donnas whose ego is dented by having a patient suggest a method of treatment and know compelling reasons for its use. Even those will probably be willing to report your bad and good fractions to you. You know the guidelines for treatment: LDLC (bad) below 100 in those with heart attack or other previous event, below 130 for everyone else; HDLC 45 or higher for everyone.

If your doctor knows that your cholesterol fractions are not within those guidelines and chooses not to treat this problem, ask him why. He may have a good reason. In the medical section you will learn a few reasons which might lead a physician not to treat undesirable cholesterol fractions, especially in some of their elderly patients. If the doctor says he won't treat because he follows the ACP (American College of Physicians) recommendations, give him a break. He is only guilty of being poorly informed or having bad judgment. (We will also discuss this in the medical section.) Tell him that you prefer to be treated by the NCEP guidelines.

If your doctor is not good at niacin now (and very few are), he should welcome the opportunity to learn this skill in just a couple evenings of reading. If he does not and your fractions are not in target range, my best advice is simple: *change doctors!* Change doctors? Of course! Your life is at stake.

Before changing, however, trying to reason with him is worthwhile. Show him some of the important facts about niacin you have learned and invite him to read how easy it is to handle the drug skillfully. Most doctors do not know that EP NA exists and are still using old-fashioned unmodified niacin. Some think TRNA preparations are toxic and must be avoided. You know by now that this is not true. Many do not know that there are differences between the various TRNA products; therefore, they don't know why Enduracin and Slo-Niacin should be preferred to all others.

Let's organize the information you want to present. There's so much that you should probably not try to talk to him about it. Write it out as a letter. Then he can't become impatient because of lack of time and interrupt an oral presentation. Use your own words if you wish, but I'll give you a number of paragraphs you could use. Depending on your situation, some of them might not apply. In my sample letter, I'll number the paragraphs to make it easier to discuss them, but you'll omit the numbers.

Dear Dr. Goodfriend:

1) I have just read the popular book, *Cholesterol Control Without Diet! The Niacin Solution*, and have been impressed with the case its author makes for considering niacin the *only* drug of first choice for treatment of abnormalities in cholesterol fractions, bad and good. As you may know, the author pioneered the use of niacin in cholesterol control in the U.S. more than 40 years ago and speaks from all those years of research and clinical experience.

2) To let me know where I stand, may I have the most recent results of my bad and good cholesterol fractions (LDLC and HDLC)? If you have obtained only total cholesterol (TC) and not the fractions, I would like to have a fasting blood sample drawn for TC, LDLC, and HDLC. From the book I know that the fractions are more important than the TC. I also know what levels are desirable and which need to be treated.

3) If my cholesterol levels require treatment, *I would like you to read the book*, be good at niacin, and use it for me. We can avoid flushing by using time-release niacin and taking one aspirin (325 mg) each morning. The book tells which time-release niacin (TRNA) preparations are preferred and why. If plain niacin (NA) is advisable, especially to increase low HDLC, a relatively new product, Endurance Products Plain Niacin (EP NA) minimizes or eliminates the flush by dissolving in about 50 minutes instead of three to five minutes, as old-fashioned unmodified niacin does. The book explains how to start each type of niacin and adjust the dosage.

4) As you may be aware, *niacin does everything right*: reduces total cholesterol and bad cholesterol, increases good cholesterol, and reduces triglycerides if they are an issue. It accomplishes all these goals in the presence of an ordinary American diet. You don't have to diet to control cholesterol! Of course, I realize that weight control is another matter; the only measure that accomplishes this goal is control of calories. The book explains why diet is a weak and often ineffective measure for cholesterol control. So does another book, *Coronary Heart Disease: The Dietary Sense and Nonsense*, for which Dr. Parsons wrote the final chapter.

5) Niacin reduces the incidence of heart attacks, strokes and related events, cardiovascular surgery, cardiovascular hospitalization, and all hospitalization. But what sets niacin apart from the other drugs for cholesterol control is that is does several things which *none of them* does. These are: increase the HDL_2/HDL_3 ratio, convert small-particle LDLC to large-particle LDLC, and reduce Lp(a). It doesn't matter that these factors are not measured in clinical practice; you *know* they happen when you use niacin. No other cholesterol-control drug accomplishes *any* of these things, thus reducing these newly discovered risk factors for coronary disease.

6) You are treating my cholesterol problem with _____. The book points out that resins, besides having disagreeable side effects and interfering with absorption of other drugs, do not improve HDLC or triglycerides. They are also expensive. It says that gemfibrozil (Lopid) does not help TC or LDLC, does not raise HDLC as well as EP NA does, and, according to FDA, should be stopped in two months if the goals of treatment are not reached. The book tells that the "statins," which cost six to ten times as much as niacin preparations, do not help HDLC or triglycerides. Because they are relatively new, investigators are still discovering new adverse effects—in contrast with niacin's safety record of more than 40 years, which NCEP (National Cholesterol Education Program) emphasizes. I would prefer to take a time-proven drug with niacin's distinctive advantages. This is why I am going to the trouble of presenting my request to you in this way.

7) In its section for doctors, the book discusses these and other details you will understand better than I do, but the whole book is written in plain words for anyone to read. It emphasizes repeatedly that *niacin is not a do-it-yourself drug*; it requires *knowledgeable medical supervision.*

8) With this letter I am giving you a copy of the book. Please read it (which will probably take you only an evening or two), become good at niacin, and use that knowledge to take care of my cholesterol problem. I will appreciate it.

Your grateful patient,

What doctor would not respond favorably to such a respectful, yet knowledgeable and reasonable request? You may want to drop or change parts of the letter. In paragraph 1, omit the sentence about my pioneering work if it bothers you. I included it, not for reasons of ego but for credibility—since my name is not exactly a household word. You will omit paragraph 6 if you are not receiving another cholesterol-control drug now, or in the unlikely event that you are receiving a drug not mentioned there.

And what if your doctor rejects your suggestion, won't even read the book and discuss your request for niacin from one who knows how to use it? You decide. I have already told you what my advice would be. If you have had a heart attack or other evidence of artery blockage or narrowing, you would be foolish to stick with some one who leaves your LDLC above the recommended target zone, 100 or less, or your HDLC below 40 to 45. You have learned that only *insulin-dependent* diabetes should not be treated with niacin; a knowledgeable doctor can use the drug for milder forms of diabetes, controlled by diet or diet plus oral medication. Persons who drink too much alcohol or have active peptic ulcers should avoid the drug until they correct those situations, but a past history of such trouble does not exclude use of niacin.

If you do change doctors, first ask your prospective new physician about his willingness to read the book and treat you with niacin. There's no point in going from one disbeliever to another closed-minded person.

When you find a doctor who will become good at niacin by reading the book, work with him. You will be an unbeatable combination. By now you know enough about the use of niacin that you can share decisions with him and rejoice in your triumphs. He will contribute his background of medical knowledge and experience but may, from time to time, need to be reminded of something you recall from the book that he may have missed or forgotten. Remember that no doctor, even though he has used niacin before, will be as skilled in its use as he should be if he has not read this book.

Besides sharing your knowledge of the book with your physician, you have the responsibility of spreading its message to your family and friends. Who needs this book? Everyone, really:

- 29 million Americans with cholesterol patterns (bad and good fractions) which should be treated, by the latest guidelines

- Every person who has already had a heart attack, coronary artery surgery, angioplasty or other artery procedure, stroke, or surgery on neck or leg arteries

- Every close relative of persons who have had heart attack, stroke, or other problem just listed

- Every adult who does not know his/her bad and good cholesterol fractions

- Every doctor who does not know how important it is to be good at niacin

- Every pharmacist who may be asked to advise patients

- Persons with excellent cholesterol patterns who are dieting when they don't need to be

- Persons dieting for cholesterol problems but not tested to be sure their goals are being reached

- Every person with relatives or friends in any of these categories

- *Yes—everyone, really!*

Finally, when you learn that some one has had a heart attack, say to yourself—and anyone else who will listen—"That was preventable." Remember that the day has arrived when we should consider a heart attack or other artery-blocking catastrophe as a medical failure. The same holds true for such last-ditch surgical interventions as coronary bypass grafts, angioplasty, stents, atherectomy, and the like. For some persons it may be too late to prevent life-threatening or disabling complications, but for many it may not be.

Quitting a pack-a-day smoking habit returns the doubled risk of heart attack and stroke to a normal risk, so it really cuts the risk in half. Careful control of high blood pressure substantially reduces the risk of stroke and heart attack. And keeping bad and good cholesterol in their target ranges does everything one can do to reduce the risk of all vascular diseases. If the drug used is niacin, the patient receives the benefits of those several distinctive things niacin does but none of the other drugs can do.

Does it work? In my Scottsdale practice (since 1978) the number of my patients who had heart attacks has been *less than one every two years.* My Madison years (1956-1973) were similar, with very few heart attacks or sudden deaths in patients receiving niacin. The Madisonian with sky-high cholesterol levels and cardiovascular disease (coronary and legs) by age 46 who died of pneumonia while hosting an alumni tour in London at age 83 is a striking example. So is the Arizona painter who had lost a leg and had been told nothing could help the circulation in the other, who is still climbing ladders and painting houses several years later. Most of the stories are not so dramatic; they are just ordinary people taking the niacin doses needed to keep lipoprotein cholesterol fractions in desirable ranges and going along year after year without any vascular events.

Finding a doctor who is good at niacin can save your life. This book tells you how to find one. It may be your present doctor—if he is willing to read the book and learn. Now join your doctor and me as we review, in the Medical Section, some important things about use of niacin and cholesterol control in general.

CHAPTER TEN

Evaluating Medical Articles in Newspapers and Medical Journals

Until now this book has been written primarily for the patient but also intended for the physician. The medical section, which follows, written for the doctor, is also aimed at the lay reader who wants more detailed medical information. Both are written in plain words for everyone to understand. This chapter may serve as a bridge between the two parts of the book. It involves both types of reader as they approach medical-related articles in the news media and physicians as they encounter the flood of information in medical journals.

All readers need to know this: Just because a newspaper prints a story which, in essence, says, "A study has shown..." does not mean that the findings and conclusions are valid. Sometimes the study is flawed, but the media doesn't know this, so it prints or broadcasts the news release it was given. My warning to the reader is not to accept such a pronouncement at face value until you think it over and perhaps learn more about it.

For the patient, what to do is easy. Clip the story and ask your doctor about it. For doctors, our best recourse is to look up the original article. Many studies are based on articles in current issues of the *Journal of the American Medical Association (JAMA)* or *The New England Journal of Medicine.* These journals have been most successful at getting press releases into newspapers and onto television and radio. Both are available in even the smallest hospital libraries. Releases by organizations like American Heart Association (AHA) regarding papers presented at their meetings are more difficult to track down because they have not yet been published, and we have no way of knowing where and when they will appear.

Is It Good Evidence?

Edgar Allen, M.D., my chief on Mayo Clinic's Peripheral Vascular Service at the time the niacin idea fell into my lap, often used stories to illustrate bits of wisdom. He taught us a basic truth, which applies to medical publications as well as many other things in life: *All evidence is not good evidence.*

As Dr. Allen explained it, a farmer had some friends in for dinner and, in the pre-dinner social hour, began bragging about one of his hens, which he claimed had exceptional intelligence. He told them that while he was working in the fields near a railroad line that ran across his property, a chicken flew up to his shoulder and untied the red bandanna handkerchief from around his neck. It then ran and flew over to the railroad tracks as a train was approaching. Waving the bandanna back and forth, the hen flagged the train to a stop. When the engineer got out and walked to the place where the chicken was standing, he found that the rails had come apart. The hen had saved the train from derailment and a potentially serious accident.

Sensing that his friends were listening with more than a little skepticism, the farmer offered to prove the story to them. To do so, he grabbed a flashlight and led them to the henhouse. It was growing dark, and the hens were at roost. After shining the light around, he focused it on one large hen and proudly announced, "If you don't believe it, *there's the chicken!*"

"All evidence is not good evidence," Dr. Allen repeated, underlining the moral of the tale.

Another story, which sometimes comes to mind when I look at research reports, concerns a man who liked to drink. One night he drank only bourbon and water. The next morning he had a bad headache. On his next night out, he drank only Scotch and water. Again a bad headache. On a third occasion, after drinking only brandy and water, he awoke with a headache just as severe. In evaluating his experience, he felt that he had performed a controlled experiment. The *common factor*, he reasoned, was the *water*, so it must have caused his headaches.

I often think of that fable when some one reports a study that looks at only one variable while ignoring other factors which could have affected the results.

At First Glance

When I look at a medical article, a number of things happen automatically to begin my appraisal of its value. I suspect many other

130

physicians go through similar thought processes. You ask yourself: *Who did the study?* Some authors command respect because of their stature in the field, like Ray Gifford and Norman Kaplan in hypertension. Sometimes the institutional affiliation gives credibility: Mayo Clinic, Harvard, Cleveland Clinic, and many of the leading universities fall into this category—although there can be exceptions.

What Were They Looking For?

One has to ask what the authors were looking for. Often you tend to find what you are looking for. The writings of Ancel Keys, Ph.D. (University of Minnesota) and associates in the 1950's appeared to examine the typical diet of an entire country (quite a trick!) and correlate it with that country's death rate from coronary disease. Never mind that it is impossible to characterize an entire country's diet, based on food purchased. Never mind that death certificates are an inaccurate way to assess causes of death, worse in Europe than in U.S., where we think we have a fairly good reporting system but must admit that the cause of death on many certificates is a guess. When estimates of total calories and fat calories seemed to correlate with the rate of death from heart attacks, the author(s) found exactly what they had set out to find. They did so by looking at only one variable while ignoring many others. Other observers would come later along to point out that the rate of heart attacks was also correlated with the numbers of toilets, automobiles, or television sets— in fact, anything having to do with the general standard of living. But if you look at one factor (diet), however inaccurate its assessment might be, you are likely to find what you looked for.

Over the years when, in talks, I have used the pseudoscientific reports of Ancel Keys about the estimated food intake (buying habits) and supposed causes of death (from certificates) as examples of "all evidence is not good evidence," I have been careful to point out that Ancel has a villa on the Mediterranean and I don't.

Another example of finding what you are looking for is the study at least three decades ago in which an observer reviewed heart attack rates in men working on London's double-deck buses, specifically comparing the man who sat constantly, driving the bus, with the man taking tickets, who was more or less in constant motion, walking in the aisles and using the stairs. The drivers had more heart attacks. This was presented as evidence that exercise on the job has a protective effect against heart attacks.

That was fine until some spoilsport came along and went back to the company's records of the uniforms originally issued to the employees. By comparing the waistline measurements, he showed that the drivers, at the time of employment, already had larger waistlines. There was a natural selection: those capable of running up and down the stairs went into that job, and those more capable of sitting and driving did that. Thus the groups were not equal at the start. The conclusion that at-work exercise made the difference was not justified. Possibly the most notable part of this situation was the British whimsy in the title of the rebuttal paper, *The Epidemiology of Trousers.*

Are the Conclusions Valid or Overstated?

Does the study really show what its authors claim? This question is somewhat related to what we have just discussed, finding what you are looking for. A good example is the alleged relationship of various types of dietary intake on one or another endpoint, as in the "low fat diet may reduce the risk of breast cancer" allegation. Such a claim is usually based on a poll in which persons were quizzed about their usual eating habits, then comparing two groups, women with breast cancer and a matched group (age, possibly other factors) without this malignancy. Such a survey does not consider many variables, some of them unknown. If the group with cancer says they ate more fat than the group without cancer, those conducting the survey might publish a paper or, more often, simply issue a press release about their findings. But does such a result really say that eating a low fat diet offers protection against breast cancer? It does not! The only way to demonstrate such a protective benefit would be to match two groups with no evidence of cancer and then randomize them to either low fat or high fat diets for many years, till a possible difference in cancer between groups became statistically significant. As we noted previously, this could not be done because people will not follow diets with any degree of fat restriction. Besides, exposing one group to a high fat diet would be considered unethical by some; this would promote obesity, of which we have too much already, and possibly even atherosclerosis, at least according to popular belief.

Another tip: *Watch for dissenting results.* While the "low fat/less breast cancer" claim has been made off and on for years, other observations have come forth and reached newspapers in recent years, reporting no relationship at all. Is it any wonder that the public is confused?

I counsel my patients to use low-fat, low-calorie diet as a means to control weight but not to expect it to prevent any type of cancer. In my opinion, those reports are efforts of nutritionists with large organizations to justify their jobs. There are far too many nutrition-oriented organizations in this country today, and I can't see that we would be any poorer if they all disappeared overnight. At least we would be spared the claims of cancer prevention and other fancied benefits that cannot be proved. If they really want to justify their existence, they should devote all of their efforts to combating the epidemic of obesity that has overcome the U.S. population in recent years and keeps increasing.

Beware the Armchair Study

We don't see this so much any more, but under the heading of "How was the study done?" is the "armchair study," one not consisting of any real research but instead examining data published by others. As George Mann writes, "During the years 1955-1965, a number of 'armchair' epidemiologic studies were done. One of the most influential was the report by Keys, which used data he found in the annual statistical report of the World Health Organization (WHO). Keys selected data from seven national reports that would show a linear relationship between estimated fat intake of the populations and the reported incidence of deaths from CHD [coronary heart disease]. However, he omitted the data from 15 nations in the same tabulations that did not fit his preconceived notion." Mann goes on to comment, "Such data selection is, of course, cheating."

Today's successor to such armchair studies is a current fad, the *"meta-analysis."* The authors of this type of study don't do any original research themselves; they just pull together the results of a number of studies on the same subject and with similar endpoints, then analyze them as though this were one massive study. The larger numbers of participants give greater statistical force to the results.

All this sounds good, but it ignores the fact that the studies lumped together in this manner are really not 100% comparable, that they were done in different locations, approaching their subjects in different ways, and examining the results differently. Selection of participants and of endpoints may have been similar but are never identical. In short, they are not one large study, which the meta-analysis attempts to forge. The authors can omit some reports based on whatever criteria they decide to set up, so the selection of data may not be entirely unlike that of Keys. Nevertheless, the meta-analysis craze continues, and the results are quoted as gospel.

My advice to *beware the armchair study* translates to: *Beware the meta-analysis!*

Who Sponsored the Study? How Was It Done?

Another important question: Who sponsored the study? It is unlikely that a study with adverse conclusions for the sponsor, often a drug company, will be published. This also has a bearing on the next question: How was the study done? This is critical to the outcome. *If a study's protocol is stupid, the findings will be worthless.* If a protocol is designed to produce a specific outcome, that outcome will usually be achieved. The discriminating reader must pick apart the methods and see how they affected the outcome and final conclusions. Two studies involving niacin illustrate this point. I will review them in the Medical Section with the subtitle *The "Hatchet Jobs."*

A story about sponsorship and its effect on medical reports, which will become a classic, occurred in the 1990's. For a long time the best source of information was an excellent review in *The Wall Street Journal,* but in 1997 the *JAMA* finally published the controversial article, so the whole matter is finally out in the open.

The account concerned Synthroid, a synthetic thyroid preparation produced by Boots, a British pharmaceutical company. For years Synthroid had been the largest selling product for persons with low thyroid function, holding its pre-eminent position because makers of rival products had been unable to resolve doubts (played up by Boots, needless to say) that their pills worked exactly the same—called "bioequivalency." My current colleagues in endocrinology had long taken the position that only Synthroid and one other product, Levothroid, were properly standardized, making it certain that every tablet had the strength shown on the label. Some doctors even tell of patients' experiencing symptoms of hypothyroidism when changed to generic substitutes, which cost about half as much as Synthroid, or less.

Boots set up a study at University of California at San Francisco (UCSF), headed by Dr. Betty Dong, a clinical pharmacist. Boots executives said they wanted to find out the real truth about bioequivalency, always their biggest selling point. They chose Dr. Dong, who had published articles on the risk of changing from Synthroid to generic products. FDA was no help because Synthroid had been introduced in 1958, before FDA required data on clinical trials for new products. Thus they had no information on Synthroid's absorption, its fate in the body, and its effect on thyroid hormone levels, which could serve as a basis for comparison with competing drugs.

The UCSF study found that Synthroid and the three cheaper drugs were essentially interchangeable. Dr. Dong wrote a report and submitted it to *JAMA*, whose editors accepted it for publication. The paper's authors concluded that U.S. health care costs could be reduced by $356 million a year if Synthroid were replaced by the cheaper but equivalent drugs. [Notice that this is much less than the billions which could be saved annually if all doctors were good at niacin.]

JAMA planned to publish the study in its January 25, 1995 issue. Page proofs were at the printer, but the article never ran. The reason: the sponsor, after paying $250,000 to finance the research, aggressively strove to discredit the research and suppress its conclusions. After much by-play between Boots and UCSF, the company decided to exercise a clause in the 21-page contract for the study which said that the results were "not to be published or otherwise released without written consent" of the company. The company used this clause to insist that Dr. Dong, her team, and UCSF withdraw the paper, threatening a lawsuit for significant damages.

There it stood until April 1997, when *JAMA* published *Bioequivalence of Generic and Brand-Name Levothyroxine Products in the Treatment of Hypothyroidism*. The same issue carried a longer-than-usual editorial (six pages) by one of the journal's editors, as well as letters from two executives of Knoll Pharmaceutical Company (successor to Boots) and replies by Dr. Dong and her group. Both sides presented convincing points regarding sponsorship of scientific studies and academic freedom, with which I will not bore my readers. The editor, Drummond Rennie, reviewed several publications commenting on deliberately withholding useful information, especially failure to publish the results of negative studies. This tends to bias the literature in favor of new treatments by printing only positive findings. He concludes that "scientists should never sign any agreements that give their sponsors veto power over publication."

Rennie closed his editorial with a vignette about his discussing the implications of suppressing this report with other editors at University of Nottingham, England. They did so under the portrait of the man who would become Baron Trent (1850-1931), who gave the land and money for the Trent Building, in which they were meeting. Lord Trent, who founded the chain of retail chemists (pharmacies) that have made his name a household word in the United Kingdom, started life as Jesse Boot. Says Rennie, "I wonder whether Boot would have been prouder of the research his company had sponsored or of the skill with which his company had protected the interests of its shareholders."

"RSS"—Really Stupid Studies

Occasionally a report appears which belongs in my "RSS" file—Really Stupid Studies. The worst I can recall was a "study" which alleged to compare the effect of analgesic (pain-relieving) medications on kidney function. There had once been an analgesic on the market, phenacetin, that caused kidney damage if the lifetime total dose exceeded a certain limit. When the nephrotoxic (kidney-injuring) effect became known, all phenacetin-containing formulations were changed, deleting this agent. All this happened a long time before the analgesic "study" cited here.

I have no idea why it was done. It was really a survey since it involved interviews about the use of pain-relievers in persons with kidney damage, comparing the use of aspirin, acetaminophen (the Tylenol ingredient), and perhaps a third agent. (I think it was done before the ibuprofen era, so that type of drug was not included.) The survey was done by phone. Nothing wrong so far. However, the group contacted was *the relatives* of people who had died of kidney disease.

The families (or whoever answered the phone) were asked how many aspirin or Tylenol tablets the deceased person with kidney disease had taken *per month or per year* over a lifetime! How accurate a picture can any of us give an interviewer of *our own* use of medications, unless that use is close to zero? And how extremely inaccurate is the guess of a relative who never really knew how much or what analgesic the departed family member used in his/her lifetime? Nevertheless, the authors of this farce listed and analyzed the answers just as though they were hard data. I can't think of anything softer or less accurate. I didn't keep a copy and don't remember where it appeared, but it may have been the *JAMA*. The fact that it reached print at all speaks poorly for the editorial staff that accepted it. It posed even a greater misinformation problem when a summary of the report appeared in newspapers. You get the idea—a really stupid study!

Did They Look at All the Variables?

Even in newspaper stories, one can sometimes speculate: *What else could explain or affect the results?* By doing this, we try to look beyond the obvious, trying to help the man figure out the cause of his headaches.

136

Who Is Responsible for This Newspaper Story?

The very appearance of a medical report, whether from a journal or convention, in the daily newspaper can touch off a wave of misunderstanding or false information to the public. Then we ask: *Who is responsible for this?* Many times it will be the sales department of a pharmaceutical company, which has succeeded in slipping a glowing report about its product into the media. Sometimes it may be just the author, the journal, or the organization holding a meeting, seeking publicity and recognition. A company with a competing drug might be trying to make others look bad. Whatever the source, drug companies are quick to use adverse findings about other products in their ads, even though they do not stand up under scrutiny.

One recent example was a report that Tylenol, deservedly the most used agent for pain or fever, causes liver damage. The careful reader of the original article would have noticed that liver toxicity occurred only in persons who had taken larger than recommended amounts of the drug. The company advises that daily dosage not exceed 4000 mg, which is eight extra-strength tablets/capsules of Tylenol or approximately 12 of regular strength. Some cases were suicide attempts, involving exorbitant amounts. Besides the dosage, two other factors played important roles in leading to liver damage: chronic abuse of alcohol and recent fasting for two days or more. (This could happen if a person had nausea and ate next to nothing for a couple days.)

The public, reading the newspaper story, may have come away with the message that Tylenol is a dangerous drug because it might, in ordinary doses, cause liver damage, regardless of other factors. The correct message is that it is unwise to exceed the recommended dose of Tylenol (4000 mg a day), especially if you are an alcoholic or have recently fasted for more than a day.

Just Plain Wrong

From time to time one spots a statement in a newspaper article that he knows, from personal experience or information, is *just plain wrong.* In January the headline over a brief review of the "4S" Study (the Scandinavian trial of Zocor in men and women with previous heart attacks) said, "First solid evidence that lipid-lowering drugs improve CHD survival." The knowledgeable reader knew that the first demonstration of reduced mortality in persons with previous heart attacks was niacin's success in the Coronary Drug Project, found in the follow-up survey 15 years after enrollment. The text of the 4S review actually said, "No previous trial of any antihyperlipidemic therapy has demonstrated any reduction in total mortality

137

or coronary mortality *during the planned follow-up period...*" Aha! By adding these qualifications, the authors were able to claim to be the "first" study to demonstrate reduced mortality, even though the CDP niacin group had shown such a finding more than a decade previously.

How Did the Headline Writer Distort the Message?

The above example also illustrates this point. Watch out for a headline that does not accurately represent the story, often overstepping its bounds. I first learned this after presenting my niacin results at a national meeting in 1957. A Chicago writer interviewed me after my paper. I took pains to say that reducing cholesterol could not automatically be interpreted as reducing artery deposits, preventing heart attacks, strokes, and the like. We hoped that eventually these benefits would follow, but at that early stage we wanted to be sure to avoid such an inference. When her article appeared the next morning, it did a fairly good job of reporting what I had said but did mention serum cholesterol and its general relationship to atherosclerosis without using the specific disclaimer I had requested. Then the headline writer did me in! The headline read something like "New drug may prevent heart attacks"—or "narrow arteries," or words to that effect. The writer had done her job well, but the headline writer had boiled down the message to what he *thought* the report said, something that would capture the reader's attention.

Statistically Significant but Not Clinical Significant

About thirty years ago I performed a study of a drug for blood pressure control for a major pharmaceutical company. After we had treated a lot of people with their product, comparing with placebo periods in each patient, their medical director called me, elated with some data he had just received. Their statisticians' analysis of the data found the changes in blood pressure we reported were statistically significant. Average reduction had been only 8 points in the systolic pressure (the upper number) and 5 points in diastolic (the lower number). Because we had enough patients and sufficient readings, statisticians could show that the observed differences would not have occurred by chance. However, I pointed out, and the medical director agreed, that the magnitude of the reductions was not enough to be clinical useful. This, with similar unimpressive results from other investigators, showed that the drug was not destined to become a successful method of treatment. It was never marketed. Statistically significant, yes; clinically significant, no.

A modern parallel is the failure of lovastatin and its clones to increase HDLC in a clinically significant manner. Apparently the company has submitted data that led FDA to let Merck say that lovastatin raises HDLC. Their sales representatives have been trained to include this in their spiel. When I asked how much of an increase, the saleswoman replied, "Up to 15%." (Most studies give figures around 8%.) For my money even 15% is not enough increase to be clinically helpful when HDLC is too low. Let's say a person has HDLC of 30, which needs to be brought up to 45 or higher. If lovastatin increases HDLC by 15%, it still remains around 35; 8% brings it up even less. This does not produce a clinical desirable value. Results should always be expressed in whether the goals of treatment have been attained, not in percentage changes.

Summary

◆ Be wary of accepting at face value reports beginning. "A study has shown…" All evidence is not good evidence.

◆ Patients should clip news stories that concern them and ask the doctor about them. Doctors should look up the original report and evaluate it.

When reviewing medical articles, some questions to ask are:

◆ Who did the study?

◆ What were the authors looking for and expecting to find?

◆ Does the study really show what its authors claim?

◆ Should I accept alleged findings of armchair studies? (Meta-analyses are the current fad in armchair studies. Beware the meta-analysis!)

◆ Who sponsored the study? (A report will seldom have results unfavorable to the sponsor.)

◆ How was the study done? (If the protocol is stupid, the results will be worthless.)

◆ Did the headline writer distort the message?

◆ Is the result clinical significant?

◆ Why am I reading this anyway? Isn't it just another "worry of the week?

Part II

THE
MEDICAL
SECTION

The Medical Section

This section contains additional information which should be helpful to doctors, but it is written to be understood by patients who are interested enough to read it. If a doctor has turned to this section right away, I encourage him to read the book up to this point, so we will literally be on the same page.

How Did We Get Here?

The first section of this book began with a brief history of the niacin solution and its progress over the years. To enhance the reader's understanding, let me explain how this book came about.

After giving my talk at the Veritas symposium (Washington, DC, September 1991) and polishing my chapter for the ensuing book *(Coronary Heart Disease: The Dietary Sense and Nonsense)*, I returned to my usual practice of medicine in Scottsdale and some leisurely writing. I had begun to write a volume of reminiscences about how niacin's lipid-controlling ability first reached me in 1955 and how that event had changed my life. Titled *Meant To Be: The Niacin Story*, it was not designed for publication. Instead, it intended to tell the story to my children, two of whom (my second family, Dana and Tyler, both born in 1976) had not lived through any of the research years in Madison. I did not think of it as an autobiography—but slowly came to realize that's what it would have become, especially if I closed with an account of all the preceding events which led to my being in that room on that fateful day in August 1955. Practicing medicine full-time, I was not driven to complete this work by any set deadline, so progress was slow.

My Veritas talk and chapter had stated one position which I later abandoned: "The FDA should reclassify niacin as a prescription drug. By substituting medical supervision for self-administration of niacin, the agency could place on physicians the responsibility for proper use of the drug." However, this would not be as easy as it sounds. The same paragraph went on to explain that an amendment to the Food, Drug, and Cosmetic Act had, since 1976, prevented FDA from declaring niacin (or any "nutritional substance") a drug, in the absence of any drug label claims. It would take an act of Congress for FDA to require a prescription for cholesterol-control doses of niacin!

FDA officials told me they would welcome the opportunity to control niacin, as well as many other products protected by Section 411, named the "Proxmire amendment" because Wisconsin senator Bill Proxmire (one of my senators when I lived in Madison) had spearheaded its passage. Its purpose was to protect "health food" stores by letting them sell products which FDA has not reviewed for safety and efficacy. I didn't care about the other products but did, at that time, favor a change in the law to let FDA control use of niacin. A few others had suggested in medical articles that at least time-release niacin should be controlled because catastrophic consequences, including one near-death, had followed uninformed substitution of TRNA for NA.

In 1992 I decided to contact Senator John McCain and Representative Jon Kyl, my Congressman, who that year ran successfully for the other Arizona senatorial seat. Perhaps I could teach them how important it might be to protect patients from their own mistakes in self-administering niacin preparations and persuade one of them to tack a rider onto any bill. It would say in a couple sentences why niacin should become a prescription drug and then declare it exempt from the provisions of Section 411. Simple—right? Wrong! I soon learned that it is difficult to get the attention of a high-ranking politician standing for election, as they both were in 1992. Admittedly, I did not pursue this effort with great intensity, as I was busy with practice and with two children in their last years of high school. Before I could really accomplish anything with either of their offices, I changed my view of the situation and abandoned my efforts. It was not meant to be.

The major factor in changing my mind on the prescription-drug issue was a phone conversation with Robert Kowalski, author of the 1987 best seller, *The 8-Week Cholesterol Cure*. Just about everyone knows there's no such thing, but the title managed to sell a lot of books. I had not read the book but was aware that it recommended diet, oat bran (remember the oat bran craze?), and niacin. ("One out of three isn't bad, Bob," I told him after we became acquainted.) I also knew that the niacin preparation he advised was

Endur-acin, about which I had also heard from a Phoenix area physician, Glenn Friedman, who shared my interest in cholesterol control and was applying his knowledge by offering coronary risk screening and control of risk factors to businesses. I did not use Endur-acin, however, because at that time the product had to be ordered by mail from the company, which I considered an indignity I would not ask of my patients. In recent years I have learned that the Endurance Products mail-order operation is smooth, fast, and cheap—showing me how wrong early assumptions can be.

In 1992 a Scottsdale colleague gave me his copy of the Kowalski book. For the first time I paged through it. I can't recall how or why I first contacted the author, but since then we have had a friendly if infrequent correspondence and a few phone calls. In one of these calls I mentioned my feeling about changing the law to permit control of niacin as a prescription drug. Bob disagreed, pointing out that FDA might insist on more studies to define the release patterns from various preparations or more safety studies. Anything of this sort would put some producers out of business and raise the price of niacin products for everyone. How could we be sure that the greedy manufacturers of the expensive drugs would not bring pressure for more and more studies, trying to eliminate niacin as a competing product?

Kowalski convinced me that the preferable course would be to leave things as they are, with no added regulation, but to educate the public (along with the medical profession) in the proper use of niacin, including the necessary safeguards. This would mean teaching the public that niacin is not a do-it-yourself drug, that it requires knowledgeable medical supervision. It would mean sharing with all doctors (and their patients) what I know about niacin after using it for more than 40 years. This book is the result, but it didn't come immediately or easily.

In June 1996 I copyrighted a manuscript of more than 400 double-spaced typed pages. As a book, it would have been more than 300 pages long. I tried to document the contributions of many medical authors and groups, giving the physician-reader a broad background in this field. In the introduction I said the book was not encyclopedic, but it came close. It devoted a chapter to each of the side effects and potential problems, quoting medical articles and commenting on them. There was a chapter on infrequent (and sometimes incorrect) side effects attributed to the drug. Another chapter reviewed papers on niacin in recent years, including some designed to show it in a bad light by comparing it to statins on an unlevel playing field. A chapter on other drugs spent too much space on several agents which are no longer on the market, a part of my historical recollection from long years of work in this field, with no practical value to today's patients or their doctors. In following discussions I shall refer to this 1996-copyrighted but unpublished manuscript as "the long book."

The next to last chapter of the book was the longest; it would have filled nearly 50 printed pages. Titled *Where Are We Now and Where Should We Be Going?*, it was a series of questions and answers I considered important as we examine our ability to prevent heart attacks and other cardiovascular events. Some of these matters, greatly condensed, are in this section. Their message, in a nutshell: We are not using what we know to be of proven value. Let's concentrate on bringing known benefits to those who are not receiving them, while keeping an eye on other methods that may eventually prove to be helpful but on which the jury is still out. And let's try to simplify life for everyone instead of making it more complicated. The best example of this is not to waste time trying to control cholesterol problems with dietary methods, which are ordinarily not effective; instead, get right to all of niacin's important benefits, in the hands of a skilled doctor with an informed patient.

The Common Misconceptions

When explaining the use of niacin to doctors, I try to start by shattering the common misconceptions that have kept them from using the drug at all, or from using it successfully (if they have tried it without the skills taught in this book). Some of these have been discussed in earlier chapters, but let's list them and comment briefly.

Misconception #1:

Niacin causes an intolerable flush. Often a physician has this misconception because he has tried one or two patients on plain niacin (NA) without really knowing how to manage the drug or his patient. When a patient calls with an uncomfortable flush from the first dose, he feels sympathetic, tells her to stop the drug, and develops a prejudice against it. My reader knows by now that flushing can be avoided by using aspirin (325 mg) each morning and by starting treatment with time-release niacin (TRNA). If the doctor prefers NA rather than TRNA, flushing can be minimized by the morning aspirin and by using intermediate-release Endurance Products Plain Niacin (EP NA) instead of the old-fashioned unmodified niacin. If the doctor chooses either NA or EP NA to start treatment, the flush will go away in a short time, usually a few days, if the initial dose is 1000 mg three times a day, with meals. Starting lower and increasing the dose more slowly usually prolongs the flush.
146

Misconception #2:

Niacin is hazardous because it causes toxic effects to the liver. In skilled hands (a physician good at niacin, with a cooperative patient) this does not need to cause concern. The skillful doctor knows the important difference in managing dosages of NA and TRNA. He makes sure the patient knows the rules to avoid liver troubles: Do not change preparations or dose without the physician's approval. Report illness and have liver tests if advised. A doctor good at niacin knows that mild elevations of liver enzyme test results are a normal part of niacin therapy in some patients and should be ignored. If the enzyme values exceed two to three times the upper limits of normal, they are significant but will promptly return to normal when niacin is stopped.

Misconception #3:

The medical literature is filled with reports of adverse effects of niacin on the liver, even some controlled studies showing toxic effects in higher doses of TRNA. This requires more than a paragraph to refute. Let me abridge my chapter on liver effects from the long book. In short, the message is:

1) Over more than 40 years, there have been only 18 reported cases of liver toxicity. Some of them have questionable features. A few have been very serious. Most, if not all, could have been avoided by knowledgeable management.

2) There have been two "hatchet jobs" in recent years, designed to make niacin look bad. They do not stand up to scrutiny by the knowledgeable reader.

Changes in Hepatic Function Tests: Significance and Management

That erudite title headed a chapter which would have been about 32 pages long if the long book had been published. The chapter began by recounting our early discovery of abnormal liver function tests after a couple years of niacin studies, coinciding with trials of early time-release products in Madison and at the Mayo Clinic. By studying these changes intensively, I eventually came to the conclusion that the ordinary changes in liver enzymes represented temporary alterations in liver function but were not associated with damage to liver tissue, recognizable by microscopic examination of biopsied liver tissue. I reported my findings and reasoning in two back-to-back articles in the *Archives of Internal Medicine* in 1961 and in a chapter in

Rudolf Altschul's book in 1964. The main evidence for my conclusions was summarized in six points:

1) The abnormalities in hepatic function are most frequent in tests of enzymatic function—SGOT, SGPT, LDH, and alkaline phosphatase, in that approximate order of frequency.

2) Several sustained-release preparations, used experimentally and never commercially available, had produced a considerably greater incidence of upper gastrointestinal irritation (nausea) and hepatic dysfunction than plain niacin.

3) The observed biochemical abnormalities were rapidly reversible after discontinuation of therapy or after replacement of time-release niacin with plain niacin.

4) No consistently abnormal pattern had been found in liver biopsies in patients with the most abnormal liver function studies.

5) Normal hepatic histology [microscopic anatomy] had been found in seventeen patients who volunteered to have liver biopsies after one year of niacin therapy and in five patients with abnormal liver function tests after treatment for intervals ranging from three weeks to five and a half years of treatment.

6) Patients with abnormal liver function tests had subsequently taken plain niacin for prolonged periods without further evidence of hepatic dysfunction.

With hindsight (more than three decades later) I can critique my own reasoning of 1961. The evidence just listed applies to the mild, nonprogressive changes in hepatic function tests; it does not apply to significant elevation of enzymes two to three times normal levels. We have already discussed this distinction.

Absence of Liver Problems in the Coronary Drug Project

The CDP (1966-1974) furnished a major demonstration of niacin's safety as regards the liver. Of its 7,700 men with at least one prior heart attack, 1,100 men were started on niacin and followed for at least five years. In the chapter on management of niacin's side effects, I explained the careful CDP protocol for investigating any possible adverse effects on the liver. None of the CDP drugs caused liver damage. A few participants had abnormal function tests and liver biopsies, not only with niacin but the other study drugs as well. All were due to alcohol.

Case Reports of Liver Toxicity in the Medical Literature

In reviewing medical literature for the long book, I found only 18 case reports documenting significant liver toxicity over the years. Abnormal liver tests, even if accompanied by nausea (which some authors like to call "hepatitis"), were not counted if the report showed a rapid return to normal when niacin was discontinued and if the case had no other distinctive features. Only 18 cases in more than 40 years of a drug's use is really not bad, especially since many of the cases clearly could have been prevented by knowledgeable management. One must remember also the use of niacin has greatly increased in the last two decades. The three factors most responsible for this increase have been the CDP results (1975) and subsequent survival survey (1986), Kowalski's 1987 book, and the NCEP guidelines (1988, 1993).

Without laboring each case report at length, as in the long book's chapter, I think it is useful just to mention what various authors have reported and what their cases teach the reader. As usual, when medical terms are used, I will parenthetically explain them for the nonmedical reader. I don't think doctors will be insulted.

◆ In 1969, Kohn (Buffalo) reported liver damage in a man who had been taking the intermediate-release preparation aluminum nicotinate, then on the market as Nicalex. His dose, fairly high (3.0 g a day) but not outlandish, had been given for four years. He developed intrahepatic obstructive jaundice, the kind so often shown by drugs like Thorazine, which was then quite popular. All of the findings reverted to normal when the drug was stopped. A needle biopsy of the liver showed "intrahepatic cholestasis" [back-up of bile in ducts within the liver], "portal chronic inflammation" [in the area often damaged by alcohol], and fibrosis [scar tissue, a common finding in alcoholic cirrhosis].

Kohn's patient died two years later of coronary occlusion, having received no more niacin in any form. At autopsy the liver looked normal to the naked eye but still showed fibrosis resembling the type of cirrhosis that follows viral hepatitis. The authors may have been correct in attributing some of the liver changes to niacin, especially since chemical findings reversed promptly when they stopped the drug, but it is likely that other factors [either virus or alcohol] contributed to the observed liver damage, which was not the cause of death.

◆ In 1975 Einstein and associates (Boston) reported a case of jaundice blamed on niacin, but certain atypical features suggest that other factors may have played a part. A 22-year-old woman had been taking niacin 3.0 g per day for two and a half years, along with large doses of several vitamin preparations "for a psychologic disturbance." She became jaundiced and itchy [the latter not usual with drug-induced jaundice], saw her doctor two weeks later, and was hospitalized. Although niacin was stopped on admission, liver tests were still abnormal on Day 5, so liver biopsy was done. The sample showed acute hepatitis with "submassive necrosis [tissue death] and marked cholestasis [back-up of bile in ducts within the liver]. By Day 11, she felt better, her liver tests showed definite improvement, and she left the hospital. On Day 38, the liver tests showed only mildly abnormal values but subsequently returned to normal. The authors correctly commented on the unusually slow return to normal of the liver tests. They should also have registered surprise about the very unusual occurrence of trouble after two and a half years on a relatively small dose of plain niacin. One wonders whether other unknown factors might have been overlooked in this young woman with a psychologic disturbance.

◆ In 1983 Patterson and associates (Houston) reported a 41-year-old man with loss of appetite, nausea, vomiting, dull abdominal pain and low back pain, then jaundice and itching. He had been self-administering niacin (4.5 g per day) along with large doses of niacinamide and other B vitamins. His SGOT and SGPT levels were very high (2,660 and 3,300 units—normals less than 50). Bilirubin was high, consistent with his jaundice. Prothrombin time was high enough to impair clotting, an unusual finding with niacin unless liver damage is severe. Liver biopsy showed changes expected in drug-induced hepatitis. Off all medications, the patient had normal liver tests a month later and 14 months later. A repeat biopsy 14 months later showed normal liver tissue. This sequence of events is consistent with my early experience and that of others.

◆ Clementz and Holmes (Peoria, Illinois) reported in 1987 a disturbing case which they titled *Nicotinic Acid-Induced Fulminant Hepatic Failure.* A 46-year-old man, taking 3.0 g of niacin daily after coronary angioplasty, showed evidence of "modest hepatocellular injury" a month later. Treatment was stopped, then resumed after six months. Ten weeks later he presented with "fulminant hepatic failure." "Fulminant," derived from the Latin word for lightning, expressed the suddenness with which evidence of serious trouble struck. His urine had been dark [bile pigment] for four days, followed by lethargy, somnolence, and confusion. Other tests were correspondingly elevated, including bilirubin and prothrombin time. Blood ammonia was 93 (normal 11-35). [Inability of a failing liver to process end-products of protein metabolism can result in excessive blood ammonia, which causes confusion and may lead to coma.] Tests for viral hepatitis were negative. By Day 3 without niacin, liver test results had begun to return to normal. Vitamin K raised his deficient prothrombin level and a low protein diet lessened the ammonia excess, as did a drug to remove ammonia. He was lucid by Day 6, with tests almost back to normal. With continued improvement, he left the hospital on Day 10. Four months later he was clinically well, with all tests normal.

The authors believed that the severe degree of toxicity developed in part from the patient's failure to follow their instructions. Niacin had been resumed after six weeks without the drug, and liver tests a week later had given normal results. They then advised him to return to recheck the liver tests after three weeks. He failed to do so and continued to take niacin "at a time when hepatotoxicity was developing and increasing in severity." They became gun-shy after this experience and advised more frequent rechecking of liver tests than I think is necessary. Something about this patient was different, causing him to have severe, life-threatening liver damage on a dose which most people tolerate without problems.

◆ In 1989 Mullin and associates (Johns Hopkins, Baltimore) reported an extremely unfortunate case that teaches an important lesson. Their Preventive Cardiology Unit treated a 44-year-old attorney with plain niacin after he had a coronary angioplasty. His dosage was 6.0 g per day, a substantial but entirely proper dose for plain niacin. In a man with coronary disease at this early age, the body factory was probably very abnormal and required this level of control. Liver tests had been normal in May 1988. In July he began taking, *in the same dosage*, sustained-release niacin which he had purchased at a "health food" store. (Although not spelled out in the paper, one of the authors told me the attorney was away from home at a meeting, had forgotten to take his niacin with him, and bought the time-release product to replace it.) The TRNA dosage, 6.0 g per day, is twice the maximum dose I ever use or recommend.

Three days later he had nausea, vomiting, vague abdominal pain, slight fever, dark urine, and bleeding gums. When admitted to his local hospital, he was jaundiced, confused, and agitated. Physical examination was otherwise normal, including a liver of normal size. All blood tests of liver function were grossly abnormal. Jaundice and confusion worsened over the next 24 hours, leading to his transfer to Johns Hopkins for management of his fulminant [lightning-like] liver failure. Within another 24 hours he was comatose despite measures to remove ammonia from the blood. After vitamin K brought the prothrombin level (and, therefore, blood clotting) to normal, surgeons performed successful liver transplantation. He left the hospital three weeks later.

The small, shrunken liver they removed showed massive collapse of the usual architecture. In the small amount of viable liver tissue that remained, back pressure in microscopic bile ducts was prominent, as it usually is in drug-induced hepatic toxicity.

I have previously emphasized that changing from NA to TRNA in the same dosage is dangerous because it has the effect of approximately doubling the dose. This case shows how dire the consequences can be. I feel certain that the Hopkins group teaches their patients the important differences between plain and time-release niacin, but somehow this unfortunate man took a very large, toxic dose of TRNA. Perhaps he did not realize he had purchased a time-release form. I have seen labels with "NIACIN" in large letters and "time-release" in small letters which could be missed. This should never happen.

Before the era of transplant surgery, this would have been a death. It should make us all redouble our efforts to limit niacin's use to knowledgeable supervision and educate everyone who takes it *not to change to a time-release product unless the doctor advises the change and specifies the dose.*

◆ Also in 1989 Ferenchick and Rovner (East Lansing, Michigan) reported a case which combined hepatic dysfunction and gastrointestinal bleeding. A 20-year-old man with depression, on a stable dose of a tranquilizer for years but no other medication, started taking niacin 6.0 g per day. After a week he had joint and muscle aching, abdominal pain, and nausea. He vomited blood twice and became weak. The liver area was tender, but that organ was not enlarged. A stool test for blood was negative and his hemoglobin level was normal, so the blood loss was not massive.

Liver tests were abnormal, but I cannot tell you to what extent. The paper was published in one of the journals which chooses to express its values only in "SI units," a language almost no one in this country uses or understands. The only reason for using SI units is to bring conformity to publications regardless of their country of origin. This may sound commendable, but it is like changing U.S. measurements to the metric system; the rest of the world might understand but Americans won't, and we have to decide which is more important. When editorial boards specify SI units and do not follow them with the more familiar *mg* values, they choose a language most U.S. readers have no desire to learn. This makes much of the material they publish worthless. Even the name, *Systeme Internationale*, is French, reminding me of comedian Steve Martin's observation: "Those French people—they have a different word for everything!"

The patient's stomach was not scoped to confirm the presumptive diagnosis of ulcer in stomach or duodenum; he was just treated with anti-ulcer measures. Nine days later he was free of symptoms, and his studies were "normalizing." After that he was lost to follow-up. I doubt that this man had an ulcer, partly because, as previously discussed, niacin does not cause peptic ulcer. It can, however, cause nausea and vomiting in this dosage range. Vomiting can lead to a tear in the lining of the esophagus, called a "Mallory-Weiss tear," which can bleed. A doctor should not try to diagnose from written accounts by those who were present, but I wonder how many doctor-readers would agree with me that this possibility makes more sense than a niacin-induced ulcer. This case report added nothing to what we already knew about hepatic dysfunction during niacin therapy.

◆ In a 1990 letter to *JAMA*, Hodis (Los Angeles) presented the first report of hepatic injury and liver failure associated with a low daily dose of time-release niacin. A 32-year-old man had taken one 500 mg "super-timed-release" niacin tablet from a "health food" store daily for two months when he developed symptoms often associated with drug-related liver problems: diffuse abdominal discomfort, nausea, vomiting, loss of appetite, and general weakness. He had jaundice, a tender and slightly enlarged liver, and a trace of blood on stool testing.

Liver enzymes were markedly abnormal: SGOT and SGPT both over 9,000 (normal less than 50), LDH over 12,000 (normal to 250). Prothrombin and bilirubin were also elevated, the latter consistent with visible jaundice. Kidney function tests were also abnormal. Liver failure progressed until he was comatose. Acute kidney failure required dialysis, and respiratory failure required a ventilator. Niacin had been stopped on admission to the hospital. The patient regained consciousness in seven days and left the hospital in ten days. Eight weeks later all laboratory results were normal except borderline values for SGOT, SGPT, and LDH.

Hodis properly pointed out that serious liver damage was possible from even this small dose of time-release niacin. It is the only instance I have encountered with severe trouble on such a small dose, which somehow had to be related to the bizarre "super-timed-release" product. This case re-emphasizes two lessons which cannot be repeated too often. First, niacin is not a do-it-yourself drug. It requires knowledgeable medical supervision. Second, all time-release preparations are not alike. Each doctor should select one or two time-release products with which he is thoroughly familiar and insist that his patients use only those. As a general rule, based on reports cited in this chapter, I would advise that patients and physicians avoid time-release preparations sold in "health food" stores.

◆ Henkin and associates (Birmingham, Alabama) also expressed concern about niacin's availability without a prescription and its unmonitored use. They reported three cases, two of them with very brief exposure to TRNA after tolerating NA *in the same dose*. One patient bought a TRNA product on his own and substituted it for NA in the same mg dose (4000 mg, or 4.0 g, per day—about twice the average doses of TRNA needed by most patients, which are 1.5 to 2.0 g per day.

One man presented with nausea and a brief fainting episode. He showed the usual abnormalities in liver tests, plus elevated bilirubin and prothrombin, which occur only with more serious liver involvement. Maximum enzyme levels occurred after two days and "gradually declined to normal during the following four weeks." A month later plain niacin was again administered and the dose gradually increased to 4000 mg per day. After more than six months at this dosage, side effects were minimal and results of liver function tests were normal.

In a 47-year-old man with a prior heart attack and coronary angioplasty, the authors prescribed plain niacin in doses increasing to 2000 mg per day. When flushing occurred in the first week, *his pharmacist* advised time-release niacin, which the patient took according to the previous plan, starting low and slowly increasing the dose. Two months later, just after increasing his dose to 500 mg four times a day, liver tests were elevated (SGOT and SGPT 155 to 160). TRNA was promptly discontinued and replaced with NA, as originally planned. Six months later, the patient was tolerating plain niacin well and had normal results in liver function tests.

These findings confirmed what I had reported in the early 1960's, that persons with abnormal hepatic function tests on TRNA could subsequently tolerate NA without clinical or laboratory problems.

◆ In 1991 Etchason and associates (Mayo Clinic, Rochester, Minnesota) reported hepatic dysfunction in five patients on "low-dose" (3.0 g a day or less) of *time-release* niacin. This statement shows that the authors did not understand that doses above 2.0 g per day, while not entirely unwise to use under careful supervision in the few patients who may need them, are not really "low dose." Dosage was 3.0 g a day in one, 2.5 g in one, 2.0 g in two, and 1.5 g a day in one. The drugs were from several manufacturers.

None of these patients was very sick, perhaps because they were under good medical supervision. Enzyme elevations were not very great. As expected, they returned to normal quickly and symptoms subsided promptly, usually within a few days, when the time-release drugs were stopped. One patient who had trouble on 2.0 g per day later took 1.5 g of TRNA daily without problems. This is the other way out if nausea or abnormal liver function tests occur: *Reduce the dose.*

These cases, which promptly reversed when TRNA was stopped or the dose reduced, do not really deserve to be counted in the 18 cases I found in the literature. Their elimination, if I had chosen not to mention them, would have reduced the total to 13 cases.

◆ Another letter to the editor of a medical journal, this one by Frost (San Francisco) in 1991, showed that troubles may ensue not only on changing from NA to TRNA but also on changing from one crystalline (plain) product to another. A man already receiving a cholesterol-reducing resin was given NA as a second agent. The dose of "Crystalline Pure Niacin" was advanced to 1.5 g a day, with the flush subsiding as expected and liver function tests normal. Four days after substituting a different NA preparation, he had weakness and nausea; five days later he was told he had hepatitis. After stopping niacin and resin, SGOT levels fell successively from 957 to normal in about three weeks.

There is nothing new here. The report merely shows that when knowledgeable doctors find hepatic enzyme levels that reach two to three times the upper limit of normal or higher, they stop niacin and the results return to normal soon, with disappearance of any associated symptoms. This one may not deserve to be counted either, but I include it because it illustrates a couple of lessons.

Frost commented that he had observed patients using "regular" niacin who presented with a triad of nausea (rarely vomiting), elevated hepatic transaminase (usually mild) and *hypolipidemia* (lower than normal levels of fat-like substances in the blood, usually referring to cholesterol). I recall in the early years (1960 or earlier) talking with Dick Achor and Ken Berge, colleagues who continued the studies I had begun at the Mayo Clinic, about the fact that at both locations we had seen a few patients with *unexpectedly low levels of total cholesterol,* followed soon by abnormalities in hepatic function tests. I don't think either they or I ever mentioned these observations in print.

In my opinion, the only discrepancy in Frost's "triad" is that these findings are more likely to occur with TRNA. The lesson in his report is that, even for plain niacin, "all niacin is not the same." A clinician choosing plain niacin would be wise to insist that his patients use only one or two brands in which he has confidence, the same advice I expressed for TRNA preparations. Since it has been available, EP NA has been my choice, for reasons discussed previously.

◆ Later in 1991 Fischer and associates (Boise, Idaho) reported a death from another case of fulminant hepatic failure following "low-dose" TRNA therapy. Their patient was a 56-year-old man, hospitalized for a respiratory infection superimposed on chronic lung disease (emphysema). He had a cough, asthma-like spasm of the bronchial tubes, and a low blood oxygen level. For nine months he had been taking TRNA (a beadlet type) in a prescribed dose of 250 mg twice daily for five months, then 1000 mg twice daily. However, a review of unused medication suggested that he had been taking only 50% of the latter amount.

He was treated with an antibiotic (Augmentin), a cortisone-like agent (Medrol) for his asthma, and an anti-ulcer agent (Carafate), presumably to prevent ulcer while taking Medrol. He also received heparin, an injected anticoagulant, the reason for which was not clearly stated. On this program his respiratory symptoms had their ups and downs for five days. The oxygen level was better, and he was eating well.

On Day 5 he had burning epigastric [midline upper abdominal] pain. A stool test for blood was positive. Medrol was stopped and another anti-ulcer drug (Zantac) added. On Day 6 jaundice, vomiting, and pain in the liver area appeared. All oral medications, including TRNA, were stopped. On Day 7 SGOT and SGPT were 834 and 654. Bilirubin and alkaline phosphatase were elevated, signifying obstruction in the biliary tract, in this instance within the liver since ultrasound showed no dilated bile ducts to suggest blockage by gallstones or tumor.

On Day 8 the enzyme tests peaked at more than 2,000. Tests for viral hepatitis gave negative results. Blood coagulation abnormalities appeared, as did Stage 1 encephalopathy [mild abnormality in brain function from liver disease, usually due to increased ammonia in the blood]. The man's condition deteriorated rapidly, with bleeding from the gastrointestinal tract and worsening encephalopathy. Liver transplantation could not be considered because of his severe pulmonary disease. Despite all-out measures to control the desperate situation, he died on Day 10.

Autopsy showed severe lung disease, with congested blood vessels around the lungs. There were arteriosclerotic changes in the coronary arteries and aorta. The stomach showed superficial erosions, often the forerunners of ulcer. The abdomen contained excessive fluid, sometimes a sign of advanced liver disease but more often seen in heart failure. Microscopically the liver showed extensive changes of the type usually associated with medication-induced liver damage, but it had an atypical feature in that the changes were most severe in the "paracentral and midzonal" areas, rather than the central portions of the liver lobules. I am not sure what that tells us.

The authors wrote that the admission findings and subsequent course suggested that the toxic insult to the liver occurred after admission to the hospital. Other than niacin, none of the medications has been reported to be associated with liver damage. Fischer and associates are puzzled about exactly what happened to their patient, and so am I. Assuming that he had been taking only half of his prescribed dose of time-release niacin at home, as they suggest, he had tolerated about 1000 mg per day for four months before admission. When the prescribed dose (1000 mg twice a day) was given in the hospital, he developed severe hepatic failure seven days after increasing the dosage. The authors correctly say, "Whether his acute respiratory illness or other unidentified aspects of his hospital care contributed to the severity of his hepatic failure is unclear." There is a good chance that in this speculation lies the unrecognized reason for this unexplained death.

These authors advised inquiry regarding current niacin use on admission to a hospital and careful observation for abnormal liver function tests or gastrointestinal complaints. I agree. The medication history is part of good medical practice. Proper interpretation of hepatic function tests and symptoms is part of being good at niacin.

There is also a lesson here for patients. Besides staying under knowledgeable medical supervision, *tell your doctor* if you stray from the prescribed dose. That level of communication might have prevented this man's death.

◆ Henkin and associates (Birmingham, Alabama) reviewed charts of patients who had received niacin at their institution from 1987 to 1990, including 17 heart transplant recipients. They found that 83% tolerated niacin well. There were no differences in the beneficial lipoprotein effect between the transplant and nontransplant patients. Eleven of 17 transplant patients stopped niacin because of high blood sugar, undoubtedly from long-term use of cortisone-like preparations to prevent rejection. Such preparations do bring out diabetes in persons who have inherited that disease.

Of 15 patients using TRNA, Henkin found eight cases of "hepatitis," all signs of which resolved when niacin was discontinued. No signs of liver trouble occurred in the 67 patients using plain niacin.

This report's most significant contribution was a survey of 20 randomly selected pharmacies in the area. To each store they sent a nonprofessional from their Atherosclerosis Research Unit who said she wanted to buy niacin to treat her husband's cholesterol. She asked for the pharmacist's advice concerning the type she should buy and its possible side effects. She did not have a prescription and, according to the authors, "was not aware of the purpose of the study."

The pharmacy survey disclosed that *plain niacin was not easily attainable*. She found it in only three of the 20 pharmacies. "Sustained-release" niacin (SRNA—for all practical purposes what we have been calling TRNA) was available in all pharmacies visited. Eighteen pharmacists (90%) recommended treatment with SRNA, suggesting that treatment with plain niacin at therapeutic doses was impractical because of flushing. None of the pharmacists considered the possibility of niacin-induced "hepatitis" important, *even when directly asked about this potential side effect.*

The authors warned, "Since niacin can be purchased without a prescription, many customers depend on the pharmacist's advice as to dose and preparation of the drug. In the absence of regular monitoring of liver function tests, the use of SR-niacin can lead to disastrous consequences." [Here they quote the Johns Hopkins report.] They conclude, "We think that more effort should be put into educating pharmacists, as well as physicians, about the risks involved with SR-niacin."

I heartily agree. The entire need is summarized in my advice for *knowledgeable medical supervision*: in short, a *physician* good at niacin! I cannot say it too often: Niacin is *not* a do-it-yourself drug. And getting help from your pharmacist is chancy at best, as the Birmingham survey showed. Supervision by a knowledgeable doctor is indispensable.

What can we do to prevent misinformation to patients from pharmacists? Several things. First, teach patients that it is inappropriate to ask pharmacists medical questions, including questions about their medications. The pharmacist knows many things about drugs but (quite properly) does not know that patient's medical condition or, often, what other drugs the patient may be taking. He does not know what the physician has told the patient. The patient needs to realize that the pharmacist has not practiced medicine (at least with a license) a single day in his life. The doctor who prescribed the medication knows the patient and is the only one to ask.

How can this book help? It can make sure the doctor is good at niacin. It also gives the patient information important to his successful use of niacin under medical supervision. And, since patients will continue to ask pharmacists questions despite admonitions to the contrary, this book can make the pharmacist good at niacin also. This could prevent the error-ridden advice observed by the Henkin group and also by their colleagues in the following report.

◆ In 1992 Dalton and Berry (also from Birmingham) reported another case of trouble caused by changing from plain niacin (tolerated well for two years) to a TRNA beadlet preparation on the advice of a pharmacist. The only mention of dosage is 2000 mg (2.0 g) a day for the TRNA, implying that this had also been the dose of the plain drug. I find the average dose for TRNA preparations is 1.5 to 2.0 g a day, so this is not an unusual dose. However, to go to this level by changing from a plain niacin tablet in the same dosage is about the equivalent of doubling the dose. In this case it was not well tolerated.

A 67-year-old woman was receiving treatment for low thyroid function and high blood pressure, as well as hypercholesteremia. She had previously had coronary artery bypass surgery. Two days after changing the form of niacin, she was admitted through a hospital emergency room with malaise and fatigue. She was cool and sweaty. Her condition rapidly worsened, with agitation and then inability to follow verbal commands. Soon she was unconscious, responding only to painful stimuli. She had low blood pressure, normal pulse rate, rapid respirations, and low body temperature. Blood tests suggested a possible build-up of lactate, which the authors thought might be explained by prolonged flushing, resulting in heat loss through the skin and perhaps the low blood pressure as well.

Liver tests were somewhat abnormal, with SGOT 363, SGPT 105, alkaline phosphatase 252. The transaminases meet the criteria of "more than two to three times normal," a rule of thumb for stopping niacin and investigating further. There was no jaundice; bilirubin was normal. Prothrombin was slightly deficient, worsening in the hospital but responding to vitamin K. Various studies gave normal results, including imaging of the head by computerized axial tomography (CAT scan), drug screen, serum levels of thyroid and cortisone, cultures of blood and urine, and tests for hepatitis B.

The woman's condition stabilized rapidly after TRNA was discontinued. Liver tests were almost back to normal when she left the hospital on Day 3—a remarkable recovery, given the severity of her problems at admission. About a month later, when she was given a lower dose of *plain* niacin, she experienced flushing and mild light-headedness. [The flush was, of course, due to taking plain niacin after a period without any form of the drug. The light-headed feeling is not usually a result of niacin administration. It may have been from anxiety and hyperventilation secondary to her apprehension, rather than a direct effect of the drug.]

I tend to doubt or disagree with the authors' suggestion that prolonged flushing played a significant role in this episode, even though the woman mentioned recalling something of this sort when she regained her senses. Flushing should have been less prominent, if present at all, on TRNA. Besides, flushing from niacin does not influence blood pressure or heart rate. I have known this since I first tried niacin in my few patients in St. Mary's Hospital in Rochester. Her overall condition was one of multiple medical problems, including coronary disease with a prior bypass, and her major presenting symptoms certainly seemed circulatory, including lack of blood flow to the brain. The possible role of niacin was suggested only by the time relationship, two days after changing from NA to TRNA. It is equally likely that a cardiovascular event unrelated to niacin triggered this frightening combination of symptoms, from which the woman recovered uneventfully with just supportive treatment.

Dalton and Berry emphasized the role of the pharmacist in the change from NA to TRNA without reducing the dose, citing the earlier work (above) of their University of Alabama colleagues, Henkin and associates. As mentioned before, this is a reason for pharmacists to read this book and become good at niacin. They can become a positive force by telling patients that niacin requires knowledgeable medical supervision which they cannot provide.

Summary of Case Reports

Well, that's it—a total of 18 reported cases of liver trouble in patients taking niacin, some of them open to question but many of them teaching important lessons. (I did not count Henkin's eight of 15 transplant patients on TRNA with rapidly reversible "hepatitis" and probably should have eliminated the five Mayo patients whose hepatic function abnormalities also reversed rapidly. That would have brought the count down to 13 reported cases.) This is not a bad record for a drug taken in cholesterol-control doses by millions of persons in more than 40 years since my first report in 1956, with ever-increasing use in the past two decades. There have really been very few reports of serious clinical consequences due to liver problems.

Adverse effects on liver function and (infrequently) structure are more likely to occur with TRNA than NA. This, however, is not a good reason to refrain from use of TRNA by a doctor who knows the characteristics of both types and handles them skillfully. Many of the problems related to the liver have occurred because of self-administration of niacin preparations or other failure to entrust the details of treatment to knowledgeable medical supervision. The greatest potential for liver damage lies in an uninformed change, in the same dosage, from NA to TRNA. Unfortunately, pharmacists who did not realize the important differences between these preparations have sometimes initiated such changes.

A patient taking niacin in any form should see her physician monthly during the initial period of adjustment or with any subsequent changes in dose or dosage form. Once a satisfactory lipid pattern has been achieved, the interval between visits may change to three months. Going longer without checking lipid levels and seeing the patient, even briefly, is unwise. The same is true for all drugs used for cholesterol control. At least the potential for drug interactions because of the P450 enzyme system, which has recently been discovered for the statin drugs, does not exist with niacin products.

Liver function tests should be performed after reaching the optimal dose of niacin, perhaps once between then and the end of the first year, then at annual examinations or if nausea or any unexpected symptoms occur. If a patient on a stable dose from one year to the next is free from symptoms, I am comfortable doing liver tests only on an annual basis. Each doctor must decide his own comfort level. The only tests needed are SGOT and SGPT (AST and

ALT). Only if these exceed two to three times normal, or the patient is having clinical symptoms, are other tests (bilirubin, alkaline phosphatase, prothrombin) advisable.

When I lived in Madison, a young elementary school principal, speaking to a PTA meeting, set what I thought was a world record for redundancy when he said, "I know I said this before, but I'd like to repeat it once more again." I realize that in this book I have broken his record. You may be tired of reading it, but it cannot be repeated too often: [All together now...] *Niacin is not a do-it-yourself drug. It requires knowledgeable medical supervision.* If these tenets are followed, significant problems relating to liver function will be few and far between. A physician who is good at niacin easily manages those that do occur.

Studies Designed to Make Niacin Look Bad and Statins Look Good: The "Hatchet Jobs"

Doctors ask me, "But haven't I seen controlled studies which showed that niacin causes toxic effects to the liver?" Two reports in 1994 deserve special comment. Together they represent a nasty phenomenon that I hope will not become a trend in medical publication.

I had been aware that the manufacturers of expensive cholesterol-reducing drugs, mainly the statins, were sponsoring multi-million dollar advertising campaigns, seeking larger shares of the multi-billion dollar market. Until 1994 it had not occurred to me that the competition for market shares was so cutthroat that a company might sponsor studies deliberately designed to show a competing drug in an unfavorable light. How naive I was! Two studies, each in journals published by the AMA, led me and others to suspect strongly in one instance and see clearly in the other that such malice might be occurring. Along with other investigators with whom I have discussed the matter, I feel that editorial staffs of the *Journal of the American Medical Association* and *Archives of Internal Medicine* erred in not recognizing these "hatchet jobs" for what they were when they published reports of studies designed to discredit niacin. The reader must decide for himself.

The first article appeared in the March 2, 1994 issue of *JAMA*, titled *A Comparison of the Efficacy and Toxic Effects of Sustained- vs. Immediate-Release Niacin in Hypercholesteremic Patients*. The authors were James M. McKenney, Jack D. Proctor, Scott Harris, and Vernon Chinchili. Only one (Proctor) is an M.D., so he is the only author who might have practiced medicine at some time in his career. Two others (McKenney and Harris) have Pharm.D. (Doctor of Pharmacy) degrees; the other is a Ph.D. (Chinchili). In a study purporting to evaluate a clinical method for treatment of hypercholesteremic patients, I consider it a serious error to have three of four authors whose degrees indicate that they have not practiced medicine for a single day.

The study proposed to compare immediate-release ("IR") and sustained-release ("SR") niacin in regard to their effects on the usual lipid measurements, as well as adverse reactions, "especially hepatotoxicity." [Instead of their designations, I shall use plain niacin (NA) and time-release niacin (TRNA), as in the rest of this book.] The TRNA, a beadlet capsule, was manufactured by Goldline Laboratories (Fort Lauderdale, Florida). As mentioned previously, beadlet preparations tend to have more problems, as compared to tablets of wax matrix (Endur-acin) or polygel matrix (Slo-Niacin). The authors also took pains to be sure that TRNA was used in excessive doses. Here were two groups of patients, each consisting of 23 adults with high LDLC levels (greater than 160 after one month on diet). One group received NA, the other TRNA. But the outcome hinged on the dosage levels of each type and the way the study was set up.

Regardless of which type of niacin each patient was randomly assigned, he received daily doses, administered sequentially for periods of six weeks, of 500, 1000, 1500, 2000, 2500, and 3000 mg! My reader recognizes that the protocol handled NA and TRNA as though they were equivalent drugs, which they are not. For NA, the early doses are below the levels used by the Canadians, at the Mayo Clinic, and in my Madison studies. Only in the maximum dose, reached in the last six weeks, did they use what all of us had used as the starting dosage. For TRNA, the average doses needed for proper cholesterol control are 1500 to 2000 mg per day. Pushing every patient to two higher doses is certain to cause nausea and/or altered liver tests in a fair number of persons. This protocol pushed doses to these high levels regardless of the lipid responses! Either the authors did not know what they were doing, or they did this intentionally, to produce a higher incidence of nausea and altered hepatic function tests than would be encountered in clinical practice, where the eventual dose is determined by the lipid response.

The authors listed as their "outcome measures" as: fasting lipid and lipoprotein levels, results of clinical laboratory tests, a symptom questionnaire, and withdrawal rates. This sounds innocent enough unless one realizes that investigators can rig, intentionally or not, both the questionnaire and the withdrawal rates. A questionnaire can include items that are not really side effects of a drug but are common symptoms in any group of persons followed for 36 weeks. [Fatigue and headache are examples. These are not usually side effects of niacin.]

Withdrawal rates are even more subject to manipulation by investigators, depending on how they handle patients, either teaching them to manage side effects and remain in the study or being quick to let them withdraw (sometimes even recommending withdrawal). However, at the excessive doses of TRNA specified in this ridiculous protocol, significant problems were inevitable.

The summary of results began by stating that TRNA lowered LDLC better than NA, while NA increased HDLC levels more than TRNA at all dosage levels. This is a correct observation, which others have reported and I have noted. Of course, the two types should not be compared on mg-for-mg basis, as mentioned previously.

In the NA group, nine of 23 (39%) withdrew before completing 26 weeks, the last period at 3000 mg daily (our usual starting dose). Most common reasons were flush-related symptoms, fatigue, and "acanthosis nigricans." Eighteen of 23 patients on TRNA withdrew without completing 36 weeks and the 3000 mg daily dose—no surprise to the knowledgeable reader. Most common reasons were gastrointestinal symptoms, fatigue, and increases in liver enzymes, "often with symptoms of hepatic dysfunction." None of the patients taking NA developed hepatotoxic effects, while 12 of 23 (52%) of patients taking TRNA did. Again, no surprise. NA is known to be free from liver involvement, especially on the small doses used in this protocol. On the other hand, altered liver tests with TRNA are almost assured by the doses used here. The authors themselves admitted, "Dosages were escalated even if no increase was required for control of the patient's cholesterol level."

Many parts of the paper, especially the authors' comments on the results, show that those doing the study were so poorly informed in the use of niacin products that they wrote a stupid protocol or that they intentionally chose to produce derogatory results, particularly for TRNA, by pushing to doses that would not be used clinically. A clinician good at niacin would have handled any of the adverse effects created by this protocol.

The authors concluded that "The SR [time-release] form of niacin is hepatotoxic and *should be restricted from use*. [Emphasis is mine.—WBP] The IR [plain] niacin is preferred for the management of hypercholesteremia but can also cause significant side effects and should be given only to patients who can be carefully monitored by experienced health professionals." The reader of this book knows that I agree with the principal of knowledgeable medical supervision, but to me this means a physician good at niacin, not a pharmacist or other "health professional."

The authors identified the "Setting" of the study [something not ordinarily mentioned in a publication] as "Cholesterol research center." At one point they said, "From the standpoint of a research center that routinely evaluates the efficacy and safety of drug therapies for hypercholesteremia, the incidence and severity of adverse reactions experienced with both niacin dosage forms in the present study, but particularly with SR niacin, were much greater than any investigational drug we have evaluated for hypercholesteremia." To which I say, why not just admit you don't know how to use niacin properly?

A widely respected pharmacologist (not to be confused with pharmacist), Louis Lasagna, M.D., wrote an editorial in the same issue, commenting on this paper. His closing sentence: "Taking large doses of niacin is not dietary supplementation, but rather the taking of a drug." That's what I have been saying all along!

My first reaction to the McKenney report was to put it in a file I call "RSS" (Really Stupid Studies). However, considering the wide circulation of *JAMA*, the potential injustice that this paper could do to the clinical use of niacin by physicians was too important to let it pass without comment. Every journal has a "Letters to the Editor" section. Over the years I have seldom written to express a dissenting view or to criticize a report, but this time it was necessary.

Calling attention to my pioneering work with niacin almost 40 years earlier, I wrote a critique, of which most of the substance has already been expressed here. In a cover letter, not for publication, I vented my frustration with the authorship and tone of the report. The article had been dated March 2, 1994. My letter was dated five days later. The *JAMA* standard letter of rejection ("many submissions…space limitations…unable to publish") was dated April 12.

Not only had I seldom written a Letter to the Editor in the past; I had never followed with a second letter. This time it seemed a good idea. I asked how often they receive a commentary on a method of treatment by the innovator of the method, with almost 40 years of experience in its use. [Almost never.] I re-emphasized the three pharmacists and one physician, the lack of knowledge about use of niacin, and the erroneous conclusions of the study, based on its faulty (or malicious) design. Add to this the fact that a writer for *The Wall Street Journal* had written an article summarizing the paper. The writer reported what he had read but lacked the clinical background to recognize the study's poor quality. As a result, two respected publications had brought incorrect and misleading information to the medical profession and the public.

I also mentioned the possibility that the study was sponsored by a drug company which had previously supported studies at this "cholesterol research center," possibly the manufacturer of lovastatin (Merck), who had sponsored earlier studies by the same group. Certainly no niacin manufacturer could have paid the amount of support this study required. To bring a positive result to the fiasco, I offered to serve as a reviewer for subsequent submissions regarding niacin—or any of the cholesterol-control drugs. "If I had had the opportunity to review this paper before publication, I might have saved you from bringing misleading information to the medical profession and the public, which can result in serious financial consequences to patients and even increased cardiovascular events to untold numbers of people."

The *JAMA* editors did not reply this time. They published no letters regarding the McKenney paper until August 17, when four letters appeared, along with the authors' response. Many journals do this: after printing comments and criticism, they let the authors reply with the last word, often making it appear that they are right and the critics are wrong.

The first, and most significant, letter *JAMA* published was from Joseph Keenan, M.D., a respected niacin researcher at University of Minnesota, and other members of his group. It is so well written that it deserves to be quoted directly, even if not completely. It begins, "The study by Dr. McKenney and colleagues is described by the authors as a 'well-designed clinical trial.' We would concur with that description if the authors would make more explicit the intention of the study, namely, that it was clearly designed to maximize the potential for niacin intolerance and toxicity. Despite their obvious familiarity with the clinical literature, they chose a peculiarly unphysiologic twice-daily dosage schedule. [I had neglected to mention this in my comments, but it was correct.] Similarly, they intentionally escalated both the [NA] and [TRNA] to a total dose of 3000 mg (1500 mg twice daily), whether or not the patient had demonstrated an adequate lipid response at a lower dose....

"The Coronary Drug Project, a study with 1119 subjects receiving 3000 mg (1000 mg three times a day) of [NA] for 6 years, experienced a 5% dropout rate because of drug intolerance and toxicity after 1 year (unpublished reanalysis, 1994), compared with 30% for 23 subjects receiving [NA] reported by McKenney..."

Keenan quoted McKenney's summary of the medical literature, which stated that "most cases of hepatotoxicity have occurred in patients taking [TRNA] doses of 2000 mg per day or more." Keenan then pointed out that the McKenney group "intentionally administer a dose that exceeds that toxicity threshold by 50%. Two recent SR nicotinic acid studies, one a controlled trial with 206 subjects and another a case report of over 200 subjects, independently reported excellent tolerance (dropout rates of 3% to 4%) and good lipid response, using wax-matrix SR nicotinic acid (Endur-acin). Both studies indicated that approximately 1500 mg a day appeared to be the average optimal dose of SR nicotinic acid. McKenney et al were obviously aware of these studies since they were cited in their article, yet they elected to design a study that exceeded these recommendations by 100%...*One must question the wisdom, if not the ethics,* of intentionally exposing patients to such unphysiologic and excessive doses of nicotinic acid, merely to demonstrate its potential for adverse side effects. Did the investigators fully disclose the intent to escalate the dose so that induced toxicity was not just a possibility but highly likely?"

I agree with these sentiments of Joe Keenan, whom I did not know personally at that time but have met since then. He expressed them well.

A second letter from Lavie and Milani (New Orleans) pointed out that liver effects might depend, in part, on the preparation used. They cited their own experience with Slo-Niacin in 300 patients, with less than 3% having to discontinue the drug because of hepatotoxicity and more than 80% tolerating doses of 1500 to 3000 mg per day. They echoed my admonition for doctors to use only preparations they know well, since all niacin preparations are not equivalent.

The third letter was from Murray Weiner, M.D., a friend from the early years of my niacin research. Originally in New York, he co-authored a 1983 book on niacin's use as a vitamin and a drug. He is now an emeritus faculty member at University of Cincinnati. Weiner began by saying that the article did not support the conclusions that [TRNA] niacin preparations are more toxic than [NA], saying that such evaluation would require comparison of doses which are equally effective. Thus the side effects of TRNA in doses of 1000 to 1500 mg a day should be compared with NA doses of 2000 to 3000 mg a day. He closed by saying, "We conclude that the [McKenney data] support the thesis that relatively low doses (500 to 1500 mg) of [TRNA] are at least as effective, better tolerated, and no more hepatotoxic than the 2 to 3 g per day doses of [NA] generally required to achieve significant lowering of total cholesterol and LDLC levels."

The final letter, from Shields and Beckerman (Los Angeles) is notable for its closing statements: "Let's put this into perspective. McKenney et al monitored up to 46 people for a maximum of 36 weeks and found no change in mortality. The Coronary Drug Project monitored 8341 men over a 15-year period and found an 11% lower mortality rate in only one group—those who took niacin. Niacin is a supplement that tens of thousands of people have purchased independently for decades. The widespread use of this substance is notable for its lack of serious consequences...Far from presenting a serious public health problem, niacin use has been demonstrated to improve the longevity of patients." I am not sure why *JAMA* selected this letter.

The reply by the McKenney group, not surprisingly, missed the point of most of the criticism in these four letters.

The more I thought about this hatchet job, the more I suspected it was malicious, probably based on direct or indirect support by a drug company making one of the statins. I was not the only one to question the source of support. A current cholesterol investigator, whom I shall not name because I believe this information was confidential, sent me a copy of a letter written to *JAMA* concerning this matter. Like mine, this letter had not been published.

The writer first castigated the reviewers and editors for publishing the McKenney paper. "Authors can write whatever they please, [but] it is the task of the peer review process to insure that statements are accurate and reasonable." Saying that studies are sometimes published because of their sensational results or anticipated lay interest, he goes on to say that a study like this that trashes a popular over-the-counter drug clearly has tabloid appeal "but I question whether its scientific merits justify publication in the most widely read and prestigious medical journal in America." *My sentiments exactly!*

The writer continues, "One additional concern, also an area of editorial responsibility is...a potential investigator conflict of interest arising from funding sources for scientific studies. When I read the McKenney paper, I looked for the footnote disclosing funding support for the research and was surprised to find none mentioned. In our experience, a study protocol of this length and description would easily cost from $50,000 to $100,000. That is more than spare change at most academic research centers. Here we have: (1)

168

an expensive yet apparently unfunded study; (2) a protocol that appears to be specifically designed to maximize a drug's toxicity; and (3) study conclusions that suggest that the FDA should eliminate SR niacin because of toxicity…I feel that a funding disclosure should be footnoted with the article, even if the source is an intramural one."

The dust from this fiasco had not begun to settle when an equally blatant attempt to discredit niacin appeared. Even before *JAMA* had published dissenting letters, the July 25 issue of *Archives of Internal Medicine*, a specialty journal published by the AMA, contained a paper titled *Comparative Effects of Lovastatin and Niacin in Primary Hypercholesterolemia: A Prospective Trial.* Five of its authors were from medical schools: Illingworth (Oregon), Dujovne (Kansas), Frost and Tun (California-San Francisco), and Knopp (Washington, Seattle). *The other three authors included two in-house doctors and one nonphysician from Merck Research Laboratories, Rahway, New Jersey*—manufacturer of Mevacor, the best-selling drug for cholesterol problems at that time!

Instead of purposely using an arbitrarily high dosage schedule to maximize nausea and abnormal liver tests, this trial chose to make niacin look less effective in lipid control than lovastatin (Mevacor) by using *smaller doses* than we had originally reported in the early literature, smaller than any doctor good at niacin would use, and not increasing the doses to the most effective levels. Meanwhile, they pushed Mevacor doses to the *maximal approved level*, 80 mg a day. This dose costs $223 a month, by our latest survey. Almost no one ever prescribes it.

They studied 136 patients with elevated LDLC levels, starting half on Mevacor at 20 mg, increased to 40 mg at 10 weeks and 80 mg at 18 weeks. They started niacin low, 250 mg three times daily for two weeks, 500 mg three times daily until 10 weeks, when they finally reached our usual starting dose, 1000 mg three times a day. The dosage changes at 10 weeks were based on the LDLC levels at 6 weeks! Maximum dose for niacin was 1500 mg three times a day. To be comparable, the sequence for niacin should have been 3.0 g, 4.5 g, and 6.0 g per day. Clearly, the design was slanted against niacin by using such limited doses.

My purpose in spelling out these details is to show how a study can be set up to make one drug look better than another by comparing doses which are not comparable. Another way is to handle niacin ineptly and play up the transient, usually manageable side effects related to flushing. These authors did both.

Most doctors reading journal articles look at the title; if the topic interests them, they read the summary, which most journals now print at the beginning of the article. The vast majority do not go beyond this point unless they have special interest in the subject. So the summary is all-important. For this paper, it read: "Lovastatin and niacin both exerted favorable dose-dependent changes on the concentrations of plasma lipids and lipoproteins. Lovastatin was more effective in reducing LDL cholesterol concentrations, whereas niacin was more effective in increasing high-density lipoproteins cholesterol concentrations and reducing the Lp(a) level. Lovastatin was better tolerated than niacin, in large part because of the common cutaneous side effects of niacin." To which my marginal note, penned as I worked my way through this paper, added "(but mainly because the planners do not know how to use niacin and wanted to make it look bad)."

By comparing suboptimal doses of niacin with full (even maximal) lovastatin doses, the authors were able to find that "At all time points, lovastatin was significantly...more effective than niacin in reducing LDL cholesterol levels." The figures they gave were, at weeks 10, 18, and 26: 26% vs. 5%, 28% vs. 16%, and 32% vs. 23%. If they had used 3.0 g per day as the starting niacin does and increased to 4.5 g at 18 weeks, the comparisons would have been 26% vs. 16% and 28% vs. 23%. They did not pursue the niacin dose to 6.0 g per day, showing their lack of knowledge in the use of the drug—or their determination to stack the cards against it.

Even in a Merck-sponsored project, they could not ignore responses in HDLC (6% to 8% with lovastatin, 20% to 33% with niacin) and in Lp(a) (no effect with lovastatin, reduction by 35% at week 26 by niacin).

The authors admit that they did not use aspirin properly to prevent flushing, saying, "Coadministration of *enteric-coated* aspirin *with* niacin and variation in the dosing to alleviate flushing or gastrointestinal side effects were permitted, but we have found the slow and progressive increase in niacin dosage to be the most effective and generally the best tolerated." [Emphasis is mine.—WBP] Instead of giving plain aspirin in the morning, before niacin, they apparently gave aspirin *with* niacin; furthermore, they used *enteric-coated* tablets, which leave the stomach before they dissolve. Plain niacin, which dissolves in three to five minutes, would be absorbed and capable of causing flushing before the body absorbed the coated aspirin tablets! Their own admission shows that they were inept in their understanding of the aspirin-niacin connection and, very likely, they intended all along to maximize flush-related side effects while appearing to try to minimize them.

170

Even so, of the 14 participants who stopped treatment because of adverse effects, five were taking lovastatin and only nine taking niacin. Four stopped treatment because of flushing, three in the initial phase; only one stopped because of nausea. Several were permitted to discontinue the drug because of symptoms very unlikely to have been caused by niacin: abdominal pain, "myalgia/muscle cramps" [!], hypotension, runny nose, and visual blurring. These are not valid side effects, either in my personal experience, the CDP, or other pertinent literature.

We knew the report of a Merck-sponsored study would be slanted against niacin in any way possible. Here's how they handled the expected glucose and uric acid increases: "Increases from baseline in fasting blood glucose levels were observed in the niacin treatment group at all time points and with lovastatin at week 18. Mean uric acid levels rose with niacin treatment at weeks 10, 18, and 26..." All this without comment. No mention that the increased glucose level with lovastatin is a surprise, not a known side effect, or that glucose changes with niacin are not significant except in an insulin-dependent diabetic, or that increases in uric acid are not significant but can be reduced by allopurinol if too high—all facts I pointed out in Chapter 7.

Only one patient developed, without symptoms, liver enzyme levels three times normal while taking niacin. Minor enzyme increases occurred with both drugs. In this regard, the authors pointedly state,"...a much larger study of longer duration (as been carried out for lovastatin) would be required to evaluate the incidence of marked liver function abnormalities." There are two answers to this attempt to make it look as though lovastatin is safer and has been studied more thoroughly. The first is my marginal note: "How about 1,100 patients for 5 to 8 years in CDP? Large enough and long enough?" The other is simply my admonition about knowledgeable medical supervision. A doctor good at niacin will identify significant alterations in liver function, which return to normal promptly on stopping the drug. We have already noted the small number of reported cases of significant liver trouble in niacin's forty-plus years of increasing clinical use.

Slanting their paper against niacin and in favor of lovastatin, the authors remind the reader: "The successful use of niacin as a hypolipidemic agent is influenced, and potentially limited, by many factors, including the familiarity of physicians with the drug's side effect profile and individual variability in patient acceptance to the known side effects or relative clinical or metabolic contraindications." That's a long way of saying that doctors should be good at niacin, which underlines the need for this book!

This article was the second hatchet job published in the first seven months of 1994. This one freely admitted Merck's sponsorship by including three of their medical people as authors. I could not believe that the *Archives* editorial board had permitted this travesty. This time, having been frustrated by the *JAMA* editors, I did not write a letter with hope of its publication.

The editor-in-chief of *Archives of Internal Medicine* is James E. Dalen, M.D., who is Dean of the University of Arizona School of Medicine. Before moving to Tucson from Boston, he had already had an outstanding career as an investigator in cardiovascular diseases. I phoned Jim Dalen, reminding him that we had met at an AHA meeting 25 to 30 years ago through an associate of mine (who, with me, had predicted that a heart attack would come to be considered a therapeutic failure). Then I discussed the Merck paper with him, mentioning my surprise that the editorial reviewers did not reject it out of hand. I also expressed the opinion that he did not have a reviewer with any understanding of niacin, the most important cholesterol control drug; if he had, the protocol, conclusions, and comment in this paper would have been thoroughly dissected and the paper rejected.

Telling him I had no desire to write a letter for publication, I offered my services to review any future article dealing with niacin. He expanded this to any cholesterol-related manuscripts, to which I agreed. A reviewer's role was familiar to me since years ago I had served this function for various journals, including *JAMA*, *American Heart Journal*, and others, even the *Archives* at one time.

Before reviewing these two hatchet jobs (articles derogatory to niacin) in this Medical Section, I expressed the hope that this will not represent a trend. However, if such efforts should recur, editorial boards should recognize them for what they are, commercially motivated ventures disguised as clinical trials. And if the editorial boards are again remiss, knowledgeable medical readers should understand the situation and perhaps complain to the journals.

Side Effects and Problems Attributed to Niacin Infrequently or Incorrectly

Having dispelled for all readers, doctors and their patients, the specters of intolerable flush-related side effects and of liver toxicity, I will now condense the main points of a chapter with the above title from the long 1996 book. Over the years there have been occasional reports of problems blamed on niacin, some of them reported only once and not confirmed by previous or subsequent experience, some seemingly valid but infrequent, and some open

07920903
SLO-NIACIN® Tablets

SLO-NIACIN®
Tablets
(polygel ® controlled-
release niacin)
Dietary Supplement
250, 500, and 750 mg

DESCRIPTION

Slo-Niacin® Tablets are manufactured utilizing a unique, patented polygel® controlled-release delivery system. This exclusive technology assures the gradual and measured release of niacin (nicotinic acid) and is designed to reduce the incidence of flushing and itching commonly associated with niacin use. Slo-Niacin® Tablets are available in 250 mg, 500 mg, and 750 mg strengths.

SUGGESTED USE

Slo-Niacin® is a member of the vitamin B-complex group (nicotinic acid, vitamin B_3) and is suggested as a dietary supplement. This product has the advantage of a slower release of niacin than conventional dosage forms. This may permit its use by those who do not tolerate immediate-release tablets.

DIRECTIONS

250 mg: Adults — one Slo-Niacin® Tablet morning or evening, or as directed by a physician.

500 mg: Adults — one Slo-Niacin® Tablet morning or evening, or as directed by a physician.

750 mg: Adults — one Slo-Niacin® Tablet morning or evening, or as directed by a physician.

Before using more than 500 mg daily, consult a physician.

Note: Slo-Niacin® Tablets may be broken on the score line, but should not be crushed or chewed.

Store at controlled room temperature, 15-30° C (59-86° F).

CAUTION

Niacin may cause temporary flushing, itching and tingling, feelings of warmth and headache, particularly when beginning, increasing amount or changing brand of niacin. These effects seldom require discontinuing niacin use. Skin rash, upset stomach, and low blood pressure when standing are less common symptoms; if they persist, contact a physician.

WARNINGS

Slo-Niacin® Tablets should not be used by persons with a known sensitivity or allergy to niacin. Persons with heart disease, particularly those who have recurrent chest pain (angina) or who recently suffered a heart attack, should take niacin only under the supervision of a physician. Persons taking high blood pressure or cholesterol-lowering drugs should contact a physician before taking niacin because of possible interactions. Case reports of myopathy (unexplained muscle related complaints, including discomfort, weakness, or tenderness) have been documented with the use of HMG-CoA Reductase Inhibitors in combination with lipid-altering doses of niacin therapy (≥1 gram of niacin per day). Do not take niacin unless recommended by and taken under the supervision of a physician if you have any of the following conditions: gallbladder disease, gout, arterial bleeding, glaucoma, diabetes, impaired liver function, peptic ulcer, pregnancy or lactating women. Increased uric acid and glucose levels and abnormal liver function tests have been reported in persons taking daily doses of 500 mg or more of niacin.

Discontinue use and consult a physician immediately if any of the following symptoms occur: persistent flu-like symptoms (nausea, vomiting, a general "not well" feeling); loss of appetite; a decrease in urine output associated with dark-colored urine; muscle discomfort such as tender, swollen muscles or muscle weakness; irregular heartbeat; or cloudy or blurry vision.

Keep out of reach of children.

INGREDIENTS

250 mg niacin (nicotinic acid), supplying 1,250% of the Daily Value (DV) for niacin.

500 mg niacin (nicotinic acid), supplying 2,500% of the Daily Value (DV) for niacin.

750 mg niacin (nicotinic acid), supplying 3,750% of the Daily Value (DV) for niacin.

Each tablet also contains: hypromellose, hydrogenated vegetable oil, silicon dioxide, magnesium stearate, glyceryl behenate, Red 40.

UPSHER-SMITH

UPSHER-SMITH LABORATORIES, INC.
Minneapolis, MN 55447
©2002 Upsher-Smith Laboratories, Inc.
All Rights Reserved.
US Patents 5,126,145 and 5,268,181.
100792-00

Revised 0903

to question. For the benefit of doctors supervising niacin therapy, I will mention (usually without comment) the suspected effects, together with the names and locations of the authors and the year of publication. Interested doctors can follow up with computer searches at their medical libraries to locate the references.

First I should point out an erroneous claim which can be dismissed by applying good clinical sense, even though it was reported by such an authoritative source as the Coronary Drug Project Research Group. The CDP writing committee for the report on niacin and clofibrate was chaired by an epidemiologist with no experience in practice of medicine, who obviously does not think like a clinician. Somehow his strong personality must have predominated over the members of the writing group who do practice medicine. The report stated that both niacin and clofibrate, the only drugs to complete the CDP, caused an increased rate of the cardiac rhythm disturbance called *atrial fibrillation*. A look at the data and some clinical reasoning can discard this as a bum rap.

The numbers say that atrial fibrillation was diagnosed in 3.9% of men in the clofibrate group and 4.7% of the niacin group, compared to 2.9% of the placebo group of the CDP. Let's think about this. CDP participants were men who had already had one or more heart attacks before enrolling in the study. Men with coronary disease sometimes develop atrial fibrillation. An incidence of 3% to 5% in five to eight years is not surprising. *Neither niacin nor clofibrate had been found to cause atrial fibrillation before the CDP*, despite many years of clinical use of both drugs. If both drugs, always innocent in the past, have greater percentages of men with atrial fibrillation than the placebo group, would it not be logical to decide that, for some reason, the placebo group simply had a lower percentage? Explaining the differences in this way, as a statistical quirk, makes much more sense than claiming a brand new cardiac effect for two well-known drugs, neither of which had ever been known to cause this problem.

There have been no other reports, before or after the CDP, of atrial fibrillation attributed to niacin or, as far as I know, to clofibrate. This is not a concern for physician or patient. In this instance at least, the CDP report was wrong.

Looking back on more than forty years of experience with plain niacin and various TRNA preparations, I find it disquieting to read lists of alleged side effects that I realize are not valid. Among these are symptoms that commonly occur in any group of persons and, to my knowledge, have never been demonstrated to be more common in those taking niacin. *Headache* and *fatigue* are good examples. Neither of these is a side effect of niacin, or it would have been apparent to me over the years and in CDP's five to eight years. I recently had one migraine sufferer who usually had a migraine every several weeks or month, if that. She had several migraines a week in a first month taking one, two, and then three Endur-acin caplets, as in my usual starting routine. Quite properly, she stopped the drug, which I will not resume, even though she might tolerate EP NA. This was the first such instance of aggravation of migraine in all my years of using niacin.

I considered the rare occurrence of *cystoid macular edema* important enough to include in the earlier chapter (7) on side effects. Niacin detractors are fond of listing *"amblyopia"* as a possible problem. By definition this is dimness of vision without any demonstrable organic defect, as in a "lazy eye." Some one reported one case in 1963, attributed to niacin in a radiologist who had been taking the drug for a year. The disorder subsided in three days when niacin was stopped. Subsequent authors have copied this on their laundry lists of possible troubles, but no one else has ever reported a similar situation. A 1991 review in *The Medical Letter* mentions "dry eyes" on its laundry list. I have no idea where this came from.

FDA, in official labeling (description of a drug's use in the package insert and *Physicians' Desk Reference*) for plain and time-release niacin products originally marketed by Armour Pharmaceutical Company (now Rhone-Poulenc-Rorer), advises caution if used with *beta-blocker drugs* (usually given for high blood pressure or angina) because niacin might induce low blood pressure episodes. Again, I have no idea where this strange idea came from. Beta-blockers inhibit the effect of adrenalin, produced in the body, on heart and blood vessels. They are one of the two first-line drugs for treatment of hypertension (high blood pressure). Their use in persons taking niacin is common since, like niacin, beta-blockers have been shown to decrease the likelihood of heart attack. There is absolutely no reason to be concerned about such a drug interaction. I have not personally observed such a situation and know of no such reports in the literature.

Other cases of problems reported infrequently include:

- Myopathy, three cases—1989, Litin and Anderson (Rochester, Minnesota)

- Reduced levels of white blood cells and platelets, three cases, two with reduced levels of thyroxine (thyroid hormone)—1992, O'Brien and associates (Rochester, Minnesota)

- Reduced blood clotting factors, three cases—Dearing and associates (New Orleans)

- Lactic acidosis, one case each—1991, Earthman and associates (Houston) and Schwab and Bachuber (Charlottesville, Virginia)

- Chest pain following unwise initiation soon after cardiac catheterization, two cases—1991, Pasternak and Kolman (Boston)

In the long book I commented on each of these reports, but here it would be a waste of my reader's time. All the effects cleared promptly when niacin was discontinued. Proper management of the drug could have prevented some of them.

The long book also contained a next-to-last chapter about fifty pages long, *Where Are We Now and Where Should We Be Going?* It was a series of questions and answers on various current issues I considered important for the physician-reader and his patients. Here I shall condense them to as few pages as possible.

Where are we now?

◆ In 1994 coronary heart disease caused the deaths of about half a million Americans, while stroke killed more than 140,000.

◆ Cardiovascular disease claims an American life every 34 seconds.

◆ In patients under 50, cigarettes are related to 80% of cardiovascular deaths.

◆ Cessation of smoking alone could reduce mortality by 40%.

◆ Only one-fifth to one-third of patients with coronary events who need secondary preventive measures are receiving them.

◆ Stroke, which costs more than $30 billion annually in medical care and lost productivity, affects about 550,000 persons annually, killing more than 150,000 and leaving most with some disability.

◆ More than 400,000 persons were hospitalized with strokes in one recent year; 20% died in the first 90 days. More than half of patients discharged alive spent some time in a place other than their own homes.

◆ Average cost for those 90 days was about $15,000, costing Medicare more than $6 billion. [Those figures sound low to me. Maybe this represents what Medicare allowed or paid, not the total cost, since they do not pay most nursing home charges.]

How many American adults need treatment for cholesterol abnormalities?

I called James Cleeman, M.D., coordinator of the NCEP and a member of the "Expert Panel," to ask the best current estimates of numbers of American adults with cholesterol levels or cholesterol fractions which make them candidates for treatment, according to the 1993 guidelines. He replied 52 million, about 29% of adults. This seems low to me. He said that about 12 to 13 million adults have coronary disease. Almost all of them need drug treatment to reach LDLC levels below 100, and only 25% to 30% are receiving *any* treatment.

How many Americans know about "bad" and "good" cholesterol?

A December 1995 survey by NHLBI explored the success of the NCEP at educating the public about cholesterol. Some of the results:

- More than 90% knew about the risk of high blood cholesterol.
- About 75% had had their own blood cholesterol checked.
- 79% knew there were "bad" and "good" types of cholesterol.
- 69% knew that the desirable total cholesterol level is below 200.

All these percentages seem too high to me. This may be an instance of finding what you set out to look for—that NCEP is doing a good job of improving American awareness of cholesterol matters.

Should we treat the entire population or just individuals?

These two ways to approach the prevention of cardiovascular disease by cholesterol control are often called the *population strategy* and the *individual approach*. They are not mutually exclusive, and there is room for both approaches. Those who issue policy statements, guidelines, and reports of "consensus conferences" are the ones who determine the population strategy. ("What shall we tell the man in the street to do?") I have always chided the powers-that-be about wanting to put everyone on a diet when a great many already have desirable cholesterol levels. This would be like putting everyone on a diabetic diet just because a small percentage will some day become diabetic. If a person's body factory and what she has been eating have resulted in desirable cholesterol fractions, she should be encouraged to continue the same program. The only way we can identify these fortunate individuals is to measure the LDLC and HDLC fractions. When we do that, we move away from the population strategy in favor of the individual approach.

An argument used by advocates of a nationwide low-fat, low-cholesterol, high-fiber diet is that even a small decrease in average cholesterol levels results in some reduction in heart attacks and related events. Their belief is based on the widely quoted aphorism, "Reducing cholesterol by 1% lowers the heart attack rate by 2%." Several things are wrong with this assumption. As the reader recalls, it was derived from the Lipid Research Clinics Trial (LRCT), the NIH-sponsored resin study for which the statistical methods had to be changed twice to make the small difference in heart attacks and deaths between resin and placebo groups look significant. With such skimpy (or nonexistent) evidence of benefit, why should that study's findings become the theme song of the "everybody must diet" school of thought?

Again, the small decreases in *average* cholesterol levels for an entire population really don't matter. Percentages never do. What matters is *whether the goals are met* in a given individual. And the goals vary, depending on the presence or absence of atherosclerotic disease. Furthermore, total cholesterol in treated patients is misleading when treatment increases HDLC, as niacin does, while reducing LDLC. This, of course, is another flaw in the "1%-2%" rule.

In my opinion, *each person should take the responsibility* of having his/her own cholesterol (total and fractions) measured, to determine the need for treatment—or the absence of such need. A doctor good at niacin can take the responsibility for determining these values in all his patients who would be candidates for treatment if their values fell outside NCEP's "desirable" levels.

The "population strategy," if any, should be to *reduce excessive weight* in the American people. The epidemic of obesity (more than 30% above ideal body weight), which former surgeon-general C. Everett Koop has decried, has increased from 20% to 30% of the American population in a very short time. Weight control requires reduction in fat intake, because of the high caloric content in fats, and also reduction in other sources of excess calories. As the population ages, obesity contributes to ill health in many ways (diabetes, hypertension, heart disease, degenerative joint disease). To my own patients, I emphasize that excess weight wears out their weight-bearing joints. This causes much disability in the aging population and much surgery to replace worn-out joints. Those operations would have been unnecessary if a doctor had taken the patient in hand 20 or 30 years earlier and helped to get rid of the extra weight. By doing this, the person could have looked better and felt better for decades, as well as sparing herself much pain.

Many people with high risk of coronary disease or other atherosclerotic problems have not had their cholesterol levels measured. A Gallup survey several years ago showed that 42% of adults with a family history of coronary disease had not had cholesterol determinations. Among smokers within that group, 51% of women and 42% of men had not been tested. *Most of those at risk reported dietary efforts,* even though they did not know their levels. We know how successful those dietary efforts are, don't we? I agree with the comment of cholesterol expert Peter Kwiterovich (Baltimore): "Changing eating habits without getting tested for high cholesterol is not enough." It is not nearly enough!

What group is most neglected in regard to proper cholesterol treatment?

Almost certainly this dubious distinction belongs to persons who have had definite evidence of artery narrowing or blockage. We have given the list previously: heart attack, anginal pain, coronary artery surgery or other procedure, stroke, or surgery on neck or leg arteries. Shortly before the NIH "Expert Panel" met to consider its 1993 guidelines, an *ad hoc* group of experts met to review the existing (1988) guidelines and recommend items for the panel to consider. They were greatly impressed by the regression studies. Their advice probably weighed heavily in changing the guidelines to say for the first time that persons with known atherosclerotic disease should have their LDLC levels reduced below 100. This was a gutsy recommendation, something that seldom emerges from consensus conferences, in which compromise is the rule and usually no one is really satisfied with the final conclusions.

The *ad hoc* group reported that both general physicians and cardiologists seemed reluctant to institute measures for cholesterol control after acute coronary events. They suggested several possible reasons:

1) Belief that survival after heart attack is unaffected by cholesterol intervention

2) Belief that surgery or angioplasty has cured the problem

3) Physicians' discomfort about providing adequate nutritional counseling [I have discussed how little this matters.]

4) Physicians' lack of time to provide preventive counseling

5) Resistance to lifestyle changes and drug therapy because of patients' failure to realize that cholesterol control is a lifetime commitment

6) Physician or patient concern that cholesterol lowering may have unacceptable risks

7) Cost issues

After a heart attack or any other situation listed above, several things need to be done to prevent recurrence. *Aspirin* should be used to lessen clumping of platelets, which can begin blockage of a narrowed artery. Making platelets slippery instead of sticky lessens the number of heart attacks and strokes due to blood clots. A *beta blocker* should be given on a long-term basis since this type of drug, which counteracts the effect of adrenalin on heart and blood vessels, has clearly been shown to lessen the rate of heart attacks. Possibly most important in the long run, these patients, mostly heart attack survivors, should have their *LDLC levels kept below 100.* This usually requires drug treatment. Niacin is the best drug.

Some surveys have indicated that cardiologists, who should be leaders in knowledgeable treatment of lipid levels, are among the worst at assuring LDLC levels below 100 in their patients who survive heart attacks. Cardiologists are busy taking care of immediate problems, doing the things cardiologists do, like pushing catheters into coronary arteries for diagnostic and therapeutic purposes, performing exercise tests and chemical stress tests, interpreting echocardiograms (visualization of the contracting heart muscle and the motion of heart valves by ultrasound). Until now they have been as oblivious as everyone else to niacin's distinctive advantages. One of my colleagues, an obstetrician, told me, "The reason doctors use statins is that they consider it a *no-brainer.*" This may apply to cardiologists as well as everyone else; give them a statin prescription and get them out of the office.

I tell patients who have heart attacks that once their program of heart medications is stable, they do not need the cardiologist; they need me. We do not need to start lipid control while the patient is still in the hospital, but it should be started soon thereafter as a part of the total plan. Otherwise, it might take a back seat to other cardiovascular medications or priorities, such as a rehabilitation exercise program. [What good is that exercise if bypasses close in a year or two because lipid goals have not been reached?] Lipids should be measured in the hospital and a definite plan instituted to recheck the cholesterol fractions perhaps two weeks later, with an office visit to interpret the results, give further information, and start treatment.

Don't get the idea that cardiologists are avoiding measures to prevent future heart attacks out of fear that they will put themselves out of business. There will always be plenty of heart attacks. Sometimes some one will ask, "When we prevent heart attacks and strokes, what will people die from? Isn't it better to die suddenly with a cardiac event than a painful, lingering death from cancer?" The answer is that cardiovascular disease will remain the leading cause of death. With proper individual and medical responsibility, the number of heart attacks and strokes will decrease but will never drop as low as the cancer rate. The ultimate effect of prevention will be people to have their cardiovascular events at a much later stage of life. I remember David Blankenhorn's prophetic musing that by reducing the development of new lesions by half, beginning at age 20 instead of at age 54 (the average age of participants entering CLAS, his niacin-colestipol study), approximately half of the men would not have experienced clinical coronary events until their mid-80's. We cannot wipe out atherosclerotic lesions entirely by present methods of treatment, but we can aim for the kind of postponement that Blankenhorn foresaw.

Here's my way of looking at it: A great many people with coronary disease have sudden death as the first manifestation. By *primary prevention* (treating risk factors in persons who do not yet have evidence of arterial disease), we can reduce this devastating number considerably, postponing heart attacks until old age in some, preventing a clinical event entirely in others. We will not reach optimal primary prevention unless younger persons without apparent problems are screened and treated according to current guidelines. By *secondary prevention* (in persons who have had heart attacks or other events), we can retard new plaque formation and reduce existing plaques, giving patients the increased blood flow which will greatly reduce their chance of a second event, perhaps postponing it forever. The same lipid treatment also stabilizes rupture-prone plaques, further preventing occlusion of arteries. We will not accomplish these goals unless every heart attack victim receives aggressive lipid control.

Should women be treated by the same guidelines as men?

Absolutely! If you are a doctor who still thinks of heart attack as a man's disease, you are sadly out of date. After all, 51% of heart attacks now occur in women. They do tend to have their heart attacks later in life. In the

1988 guidelines, NCEP listed only "male sex" as a gender-related risk factor; in 1993 they added "postmenopausal female," which makes sense. Surgical removal of the ovaries early in life particularly increases the risk of arterial disease.

For the following list of impressive facts I am indebted to a Scottsdale cardiologist, Barbara Prian, M.D., an active faculty member of the AMWA (American Medical Women's Association) Educational Project on CHD in Women. She assembled these statements in a commentary in *Arizona Medicine*, titled *An Equal Opportunity Killer: Coronary Heart Disease in Women*.

- Cardiovascular disease kills a half million American women a year, more than any other disease. Coronary artery disease alone annually kills 250,000 American women, *twice* the number who die of *all cancers combined*. Thirty-one per cent of postmenopausal women risk dying of CHD, compared to 3% who risk dying of breast cancer. Ironically, women still perceive breast cancer to be their greatest health threat. Until women appreciate the threat of coronary heart disease (CHD), they are unlikely to undertake preventive measures while young or to respond to symptoms of CHD when older.

- Women smokers develop their first myocardial infarction 19 years before nonsmokers. Teenage women are the fastest growing segment of smokers.

- A family history of heart disease before age 65 in female relatives is also a strong predictor for heart disease in women.

- Coronary heart disease (CHD) presents ten years later in women as compared with men. By age 65, one in three women has clinical symptoms of CHD.

- Diabetic women lose their gender benefit and develop CHD at the same age as nondiabetic men. Diabetes doubles the risk of heart disease in women.

- The level of HDL [cholesterol] rather than total cholesterol or LDL [cholesterol] gives the most valuable information about CHD risk in women. An HDLC level lower than 50 increases risk, whereas a level higher than 60 decreases risk. A high triglyceride level increases risk in women but not in men.

Should women be treated differently from men? Yes, in one major respect. If HDLC is too low, estrogens can be used if a woman tolerates them. For those who do not tolerate them, niacin remains the best drug to increase HDLC. It can also be used to reduce LDLC in women taking estrogens.

Both AHA and the AMWA have criticized doctors who don't seem to be interested in preventing heart disease in women. AMWA spokeswoman Anne Taylor, M.D. pointed out, "For their female patients, many physicians stress cancer prevention, through Pap smears and mammograms, more than heart disease prevention. But one of every two women will die from heart disease, while only one in eight will die from breast cancer." Her point is well taken. A 1995 Gallup poll of 300 internists and 505 women, ages 45 to 75, showed that one in three physicians and four of five women did not know that heart disease is the leading cause of death in women.

I believe that a doctor good at niacin will also be good at assessing and treating risk factors in women.

Should elderly persons be treated according to the same guidelines?

There are many reasons that treating cholesterol fractions to NCEP target levels should be beneficial in older persons, but clinical judgment says that not all older persons should be treated. I agree with Denke and Grundy (Dallas) when they say, "Treatment is difficult to justify with extremely advanced age, debilitating arthritis, osteoporosis, severe coronary disease, malignancy, or dementia." To be compulsive, I would reverse the order. Dementia is the most frequent reason that I do not prescribe or even consider lipid control in some of my older patients.

A November 1994 news story, quoting a *JAMA* paper and editorial, must have been seen by most of my over-70 patients. Its lead paragraph began, "Over 70 and concerned about your cholesterol level? You may be worrying needlessly..." In my same file is a September 1955 newspaper story headlined, "Elderly should watch their cholesterol as well." Remember my advice to watch for conflicting reports?

The National Institute on Aging (NIA) called the 1994 study "misleading," saying it "flies in the face of similar research done earlier." NIA spokesperson Dr. Tamara Harris said, "It is very hard to imagine that atherosclerosis is not the same disease in older people as it is in younger people—and therefore, the risk factors should still be the same." Dr. James Cleeman, NCEP coordinator, acknowledged that cholesterol is a less powerful risk factor in older persons than in middle age, "but there is much more coronary disease in the elderly, many more heart attacks, and there is a great deal of evidence that the elderly should not be excluded from the benefits of cholesterol lowering." I agree.

A journal can bias the final conclusion (and newspaper spin) of a controversial article by its choice of writer for an editorial in the same issue. In 1994 *JAMA* chose Hulley (San Francisco), a frequent naysayer; predictably, he supported the view that older persons with abnormal cholesterol patterns should not be treated. In fairness, though, in 1990 Hulley's group did report a 10-year study (2,746 men in a Health Maintenance Organization) which supported other observational studies in "elderly" men. They concluded that "if treatment of high blood cholesterol is as effective in reducing cholesterol-related risk for coronary heart disease after 65 years of age as it is in middle-aged men, it might actually produce reductions in mortality due to coronary heart disease."

The 1995 *JAMA* article indicating that "elderly should watch their cholesterol" was a study by the NIA. They found (2,527 women and 1,377 men over age 71), that those with *HDLC below 35* were 2.5 times more likely to die from coronary disease within a one-year period as those with *HDLC above 60*. For HDLC levels between 35 and 59, the risk of coronary death was 1.4 times greater than above 60. Total cholesterol levels above 240 was associated with twice the risk, compared with persons with levels between 161 and 199. We know the only drug that raises HDLC while reducing LDLC, don't we?

This time *JAMA* chose Dr. Margo Denke (Dallas) to write an editorial. Lacking long-term trials in the elderly, she said, decisions to screen and treat should take into consideration the patient's preference and lifestyle. [I agree—and can assure you that patients in general, and older persons in particular, do not want to change lifestyle by limiting diet severely, a measure which usually does not work anyhow.] Denke advised that screening not be done if treatment would not be considered, with which anyone would agree. She added that lipid-lowering drugs are well tolerated in the elderly, who may need a slightly lower dose than younger patients. [I have not noticed a significant difference in the required dosage with aging.] Finally, she cautioned that lipid-lowering medication may be too expensive for seniors on fixed incomes. [This applies to resins and statins but certainly not to niacin.]

Previously (1990) Denke and Grundy had reviewed hypercholester-emia in elderly persons and expressed very well some views which coincide with my reasoning. Citing the reduction in deaths by niacin in the CDP, they added that this drug might be particularly effective in older persons since it increases HDLC, the strongest predictor for coronary disease in this age group. They also speculate that using cholesterol-control drugs in combination might allow a reduced dosage of each drug. [The operative word is *might*.] As an example, they suggest combining a resin and a statin, which makes no sense. Why use together two drugs which each can only reduce LDLC and TC, while doing nothing for HDLC or triglycerides, and for which the smallest recommended doses cost about $60 a month for each drug? Where was their concern for fixed-income seniors in that recommendation? Instead, the proper strategy would be to use niacin, with all its advantages, adding a second drug only if niacin fails to achieve the goals of treatment. But first these authors need this book, because their discussion of potential side effects of niacin include several which should not be attributed to the drug (dry mouth and eyes, peptic ulcers, cardiac arrhythmias, and hypotension). They also erroneously claim that niacin "may induce frank diabetes." I have explained the correct facts previously.

An accompanying editorial by Kafonek and Kwiterovich (Baltimore) agreed that treatment should be offered to older patients who are in generally good health, taking into consideration the risk-to-benefit ratio. This is exactly what any conscientious clinician does for all his patients. The editorial writers felt that the NCEP guidelines should be extended through age 75 in otherwise healthy patients. Based on reports in the literature, they point out that if an elderly patient has a critically narrowed area in a coronary artery, whether symptoms are present or not, even a short treatment period might prevent overt disease. Quoting Blankenhorn's 1987 colestipol-niacin work, they note that *the extent of coronary atherosclerosis can be decreased within a relatively short time span (one to two years) by cholesterol control.* Their conclusion, like that of Denke and Grundy, agrees with my practice in elderly persons. It is really just common sense.

I do not treat cholesterol in persons in their 90's or very many in their 80's, but there are some over-80 patients who are well enough in other ways to make control of cholesterol fractions desirable. However, there are not many in this age group with marked abnormality in their cholesterol fractions. If present, such changes would probably have resulted in death or major disability earlier.

I think most clinicians feel, as I do, that we should not be telling patients over 90 what to do; *we should be asking them what we should be doing.*

Should abnormal cholesterol levels be treated in young persons?

The medical profession was surprised when autopsies showed some degree of atherosclerosis in 77% of American soldiers killed in the Korean War. Investigators knew, from the mid-1950s, if not before, that fatty streaks in the aorta were present from about age two. Fatty streaks are the earliest cholesterol deposits, which in time become atherosclerotic plaques. Later, fibrous tissue is added (fibrous or "pearly" plaques). Eventually, far advanced lesions calcify (calcified plaques). So the beginnings of atherosclerotic disease are present even in two-year-old infants!

A 1993 study in 111 young adult victims (aged 14 to 35 years, average age 26) of noncardiac trauma was performed to see whether atherosclerosis seemed to be declining as a result of lower cholesterol levels. The subjects were predominantly male (86%) and white (86%); 68% were smokers. Autopsies found signs of coronary atherosclerosis in 78%, including 21% who had more than 50% narrowing in places. [It takes about 80% to 90% narrowing to cause clinical trouble in most instances, but lesions around 50% are dangerous because they may rupture, suddenly blocking the artery.] Five per cent had significant narrowing of the left main coronary artery. All coronary arteries are important, of course, but this artery supplies blood to the front wall of the heart and is a major source of trouble when it is markedly narrowed.

In a much larger study, researchers headed by Robert Wissler (Chicago) found lesions in *all* aortas and *about half* of the right coronary arteries of 2,500 American teenagers who were sudden death victims. Based on these very strong findings, Wissler advised that pediatricians recommend dietary changes for children aged six and above. Mayo Clinic pediatrician William Weidman agreed with a reduced fat, low cholesterol diet for children who do not have such risk factors as family history of cardiovascular disease. He added that it is safe to start dietary changes after the age of two. (Until age two, such changes can interfere with growth and development.)

These studies showed that young Americans still have a high prevalence of coronary atherosclerosis, a good reason that interventions to prevent coronary death should begin early. But how early? And how diligently should we search for potential victims in childhood and adolescence? Then what should we do for those with abnormal lipid patterns?

The NCEP appointed an "Expert Panel" on blood cholesterol levels in children and adolescents, which issued its report in 1991. Levels tend to be lower in children and adolescents, than in adults, averaging about 160 for total cholesterol and 100 for LDLC. For children between ages one and 19, 95% fell below 200 for TC and 130 for LDLC. Like American adults, these young people have higher cholesterol levels, higher rates of coronary disease and deaths, and higher intakes of saturated fats and cholesterol than their counterparts in many other countries. [Of course, many would feel, like me, not ready to trade life styles with the South African Bantu just to have his average cholesterol levels.] Higher blood levels frequently come from families with a high incidence of coronary disease among adult members, from both genetic (inherited) and environmental (lifestyle) factors. Children and adolescents with high cholesterol levels, not surprisingly, are more likely to have high levels as adults.

The Panel suggested combining the population approach and an individualized approach to this problem. For all healthy children over the age of two and for adolescents, they advised a wide variety of foods, adequate calories to support growth and development, plus ideal body weight. They favor a diet low in saturated fatty acids, total fat, and dietary cholesterol, with "only enough calories to maintain desirable weight," adding, "The panel's recommendations are not intended for infants from birth to two years of age, whose fast growth requires a higher percentage of calories from fat." They charge schools, health professionals, government agencies, the food industry, and the mass media with the task of spreading their advice to the public.

This certainly sounds like motherhood and the American flag, well worth supporting. However, if adults will not do such things for themselves, how can we motivate them to change the entire family's approach to diet? Remember the Diet-Heart Feasibility Study? And the convincing study which showed it is all right to eat eggs?

The NCEP individualized approach seeks to identify children and adolescents at greatest risk of high cholesterol and coronary disease as adults. They recommend *selective* screening as part of regular health care *if there is a family history of premature cardiovascular disease (before age 50) or at least one parent with high blood cholesterol.* They decided that for most children *not from high-risk families*, there is sufficient opportunity to begin cholesterol-lowering therapies when they reach adulthood.

For this selective screening approach to work, children and adolescents should have lipids measured if parents or grandparents have any of the things, previously listed, which block or narrow arteries, qualifying an adult for LDLC reduction to less than 100. The Panel also advised that cardiologists routinely refer the offspring of their patients on that list for cholesterol testing and follow-up. Children whose parents have blood TC levels 240 or higher, or LDLC levels 130 or higher, should also be tested. In my experience, cardiologists are not good at getting grown relatives of their heart attack patients tested for cholesterol abnormalities, much less their children, as NCEP advises. Nevertheless, testing those children is advisable.

In studying cholesterol problems in children, I consider Gerald Berenson (New Orleans) to be without peer. For years he has headed the Bogalusa Heart Study, which has observed more than 8,000 offspring and their parents, nearly half the population of that town north of New Orleans. As in most risk factor studies, the eventual goal is to identify and treat those at increased risk.

Berenson was not a member of the NCEP "expert panel" for children and adolescents, which means NIH failed to invite the leading authority in the country to serve on the panel. At the November 1994 AHA meeting, Berenson recommended universal cholesterol screening, beginning at age four, based on his study's findings. He said that the limited screening advised by NCEP would result in under-detection of hypercholesteremia in children, saying, "We would miss the children whose parents are still too young to have developed heart disease."

Among children ages 5 to 10 in the Bogalusa Study, only 5% of parents had suffered heart attacks, compared to 25% by the time children had reached 25 to 31. Parental stroke rose from 2% in the younger children to 9% in those over 25. For blacks, in whom stroke is more prevalent because high blood pressure occurs in many more adults, the parental stroke rates were 3% for younger children, 19% for those over 25. Some believe that NCEP would identify more susceptible young persons if they included grandparents in their definition of high-risk families. This sounds correct to me.

I agree with Berenson if "universal screening" means testing children one at a time as part of a health check-up but not if it means mass screening. The personal physician is best suited to identify families who would be most likely to avail themselves of treatment to control cholesterol if abnormal.

A reasonable first goal for all children is weight control. Fat children become even fatter adults and become part of the obesity epidemic. No special diet should be used in the first two years, the period of most rapid growth. Less well known is the fact that growth failure, even nutritional dwarfism and general failure to thrive (including lack of development of secondary sex characteristics) have been reported in persons in the *first two decades* of life

187

who were subjected to severe restriction of saturated fats in their diets. Dr. Mary Enig pointed this out in George Mann's book, *Coronary Heart Disease: The Dietary Sense and Nonsense*. This should give pause to those who would advocate severe dietary modification in children and teenagers whose cholesterol patterns should be improved. The *balanced diet*, emphasized by the Expert Panel, needs to be observed. Diet may be abandoned because it is objectionable to the patient or family, fails to achieve its goals, or causes adverse effects. In this instance, a doctor good at niacin needs to feel free to consider using the drug, with appropriate monitoring, as in adults.

The need for drug therapy will depend on the severity of the cholesterol abnormality and the age of the patient. Those with homozygous familial hypercholesteremia (the extremely rare kind inherited from both parents, in which the child may die before age ten) should be treated with whatever measures will reduce total and LDLC to reasonable levels. This often requires a combination of drugs, with or without diet. Usually this disorder is best handled by a specialist in treating lipid disorders. Techniques such as *plasmapheresis* (taking blood plasma from the patient, removing lipids from the plasma, and giving the plasma back) have been tried. So has *partial ileal resection* (surgical removal of part of the small intestine to reduce absorption of fats). I recall reading at one time that a South African group was performing *liver transplants* to combat this rapidly fatal disorder—actually replacing the body factory which was producing such large amounts of LDLC. In this country very few, if any, such operations have been performed for this purpose.

The clinician must always weigh benefit against risk when planning treatment for children with cholesterol abnormalities, most of whom will have one parent with a similar disorder. I do not treat children now, but during the years of my Madison research, I did several studies in about twenty children we followed for years after their parents, adult study patients, brought them in for testing. Although I cannot generalize from the small number of children followed in my laboratory, I do have some experience in treating children between 5 and 20 with several agents for cholesterol control—niacin, resins, and probucol. There were no different problems in children from those in adults. If anything, the younger persons seemed to tolerate the drugs better. The drugs seldom, if ever, had to be discontinued because of side effects or adverse effects. We usually adjusted doses by weight in pre-teenagers. No problems with growth and development occurred. Lipid results were similar to those seen in adults.

Critics of widespread cholesterol testing and treatment in young adults (notably Hulley and associates, San Francisco) say that by diagnosing hypercholesteremia, we change healthy adults to worried people; besides, dietary treatment does not work and drug therapy is not "cost-effective." The truth is that diagnosing and treating cholesterol problems can keep "healthy" young adults from becoming dead people. Doing something positive and effective to produce "healthy" patterns of cholesterol fractions should make people confident that they are doing everything they can to prevent heart attack and stroke. Such a positive approach avoids the "worried well" concern of the naysayers. And finally, the "not cost-effective" label applies to other drugs, particularly statins and resins, but not to niacin. This is another reason for my goal of making every doctor good at niacin.

What about testing and treating young adults? Young adults are adults. They are accumulating cholesterol deposits in their arteries which will eventually kill or disable them. By detecting those with high-risk patterns, we can at least offer proven preventive treatment with a low-cost drug used successful for more than 40 years, whose safety and efficacy depends on skillful supervision by a physician. This is how they should be treated.

A View Disagreeing with NCEP Recommendations

As I was completing the long book (1996), something happened which demands comment. It reached the newspapers, where misinformation can cause more harm than if it appears only in medical journals.

The American College of Physicians, a prestigious organization of specialists in internal medicine (to which I belong), apparently decided to disagree with the 1993 NCEP guidelines. I'm not sure why. Perhaps Hulley convinced them to do so. I believe the *Annals of Internal Medicine* said that he had hand-picked the committee (in fact, two committees working together to formulate recommendations). The two members who "authored" the ACP guidelines, Garber and Browner, turned out to be associates of Hulley. A note in the *Annals* said, "This issue contains a reevaluation of the evidence by *three* authors commissioned by the American College of Physicians that has led to new guidelines..."] It also said that the committee work was completed in February 1995 without explaining why the article was not published until March 1996, despite the fact that the *Annals*, official organ of the ACP, was surely available at any time. It was not because they polled the ACP membership regarding the new position paper, which I believe would have been rejected by a majority, in favor of the NCEP guidelines.

This illustrates that it is possible to come up with whatever conclusions you desire by putting in charge some one with those views and then stacking the "committee" with like-minded "experts." The reader by this time recognizes Hulley's name as probably the leading advocate of withholding from large segments of the population the benefits of discovering and treating abnormal cholesterol patterns.

Their (the loaded committee's) guidelines differed from those of NCEP in that they recommended only limited screening, primarily for middle-aged men! Then they advised only TC (not fractions) and only once. [This despite the fact that as many as one-third of patients are misclassified by only one test, and measuring only TC will automatically miss all persons with low HDLC.] They specifically advised *against* testing men under 35 or women under 45, except with family history or at least two risk factors, saying screening is "appropriate but not mandatory" for men 35 to 65 and women 45 to 65. They took a neutral position on advising or discouraging screening for *primary* prevention in men and women 65 to 75. For those 75 and older, they do not recommend screening. For persons of all ages with known vascular disease (the "below 100 LDLC target group" by NCEP guidelines), they recommend lipid analysis (not just TC) and aggressive treatment. This last recommendation is the same as the NCEP Panel's advice—and mine.

After first reading the ACP article, I thought, "Is it just me, or is this the stupidest set of recommendations these naysayers could have possibly assembled?" It was not just me. In the same issue were three pages of masterful rebuttal by a highly respected man in the cholesterol field, John LaRosa (New Orleans). His last four sentences deserve to be quoted directly:

"This recommendation [the ACP article] is based in part on the assumption that overuse of cholesterol-lowering drugs will otherwise become a problem. In fact, a major current problem is *underuse* of cholesterol-lowering medications, even in patients at high risk for coronary events. The guidelines proposed by the College minimize large elements of the database linking cholesterol to atherogenesis and make unwarranted and unproven assumptions about physician behavior. In its rationale, its potential consequences, and the process by which it was derived, *this policy is in error and should be rejected.*" [Emphasis mine.—WBP]

Exactly right, Dr. LaRosa!

Why not rely on the marvels of coronary bypass surgery and the like?

My answer is another question: Why not eliminate the need for these heroic measures in the vast majority of people? Cholesterol plaques begin to form almost immediately after vein grafts are substituted for coronary arteries, a fact pointed out in the 1960's by Joe Borboriak (Milwaukee) and just as true today. Grafts may become blocked as soon as a year or two after surgery if LDLC is not properly controlled.

Remember, we have reached an era when a heart attack should be considered a therapeutic failure. Does cholesterol control work? Several times during my 20 years of practice in Scottsdale I have had the hospital record room prepare computer printouts, listing patients admitted on my service with heart attacks. (Any of my patients would have been on my service, then a cardiologist called; they would not have started on the cardiology service.) We have repeatedly confirmed that the total is *less than one heart attack for every year of practice!* In fact, it is less than one every two years. Thinking back to my 18 years in Madison, the record was about the same. And none of those with heart attacks were patients in my niacin studies or receiving other cholesterol-control drugs in my studies. Of course, for official confirmation that niacin prevents heart attacks and saves lives, we rely on the formal study, the CDP, in which niacin did both, despite suboptimal doses rather than individualized doses, as clinicians use in practice.

Are low cholesterol levels harmful? How low? How harmful?

Earlier we mentioned that there have been several studies in which reduction of cholesterol levels lowered the rates of heart attacks but not of total deaths, the difference representing deaths from accidents, violence, and suicide. Some have tried to connect these situations with "too low" cholesterol levels, pointing out that cholesterol is a normal body constituent, needed for various functions and is a normal component of the walls of nerve cells.

In 1992 NIH convened a Conference on Low Blood Cholesterol. Its experts analyzed 19 studies (more than 500,000 men and 10,000 women) in which levels below 160 were associated with increased risk of death from noncardiovascular disease. Among the causes were brain hemorrhage, alcoholism, liver cancer, and suicide. The whole issue has not been resolved, but the participants in that conference (and I think most observers) believe that the low cholesterol is frequently the result, not the cause, of cancer, especially in its advanced stages. The same is true of chronic respiratory diseases, another cause of death associated with low cholesterol levels. Alcoholism is capable of altering the body's overall metabolism, especially when substituted for adequate nutrition. A sick liver just does not produce much cholesterol. Liver cancer is often the result of alcoholism. Whatever psychologic factors caused the alcoholism can also lead to suicide. It is unlikely that low cholesterol leads to these conditions; instead, it is the result. There is really no evidence that treatment of abnormal cholesterol metabolism ever causes any of these dire situations.

In an excellent review of the matter, Santiago and Dalen (Tucson) state, "Changes in serum cholesterol levels much greater than those observed in clinical trials would be required to trigger a significant change in cell membrane cholesterol." They also say, "The current literature does not support a relationship between low or lowered cholesterol levels and violent behavior." And their final sentence, "The findings concerning cholesterol and violent behavior are intriguing and deserve further research, but a great deal of caution must be exercised in offering a single, unitary theory to explain the data." Like everyone else, they have said, "We don't know," but they said it elegantly, after a thorough review of medical literature.

I have already mentioned the "too-low" total cholesterol readings (below 125) we sometimes encounter in patients taking niacin. When readings for TC and LDLC are too low, often there is a paradoxical fall in HDLC as well. The remedy is simple. *Reduce the dose.* Usually lowering the dose by just one tablet a day is sufficient.

Should niacin's use be limited by making it a prescription drug?

I have already explained my conversion from an advocate of this position to one of leaving things as they are and educating physicians and patients in use of niacin—the purpose of this book. Now, seeing how easy it is to understand and manage the drug, I expect the reader to agree.

I have come to believe that making niacin a prescription drug would be a great over-reaction to a relatively small problem which can be solved by education. To illustrate another example of a sweeping recommendation for a limited problem, I borrow an account written by Martin Stevenson, editor-in-chief of *Modern Medicine* (an excellent journal of current abstracts, sent to physicians for decades). His editor's page in the February 1995 issue cited "the nuttiest idea ever published in a medical journal." In a letter to a prestigious journal in 1989, three Bronx physicians described how they had treated a man who came to the emergency room because a bottle cap had lodged in his esophagus after he opened a beer bottle with his teeth. The cap was removed uneventfully. Stevenson says, "In a truly stunning conclusion, the authors wrote, 'This case highlights the hazard of opening bottles of carbonated drinks with the teeth. *We suggest that such drinks be marketed only in cans.*' "

Stevenson comments, "Right. Let's tell the entire carbonated-beverage industry to redesign and retool all its bottling plants just in case some guy is thinking about popping open a Bud with his teeth."

Are antioxidants of value in preventing heart attacks?

If antioxidants reduce CHD at all, they probably do so by preventing oxidation of fat-carrying low-density lipoproteins (LDL) in the blood. Oxidized LDL triggers the earliest inflammatory reaction in the wall of an artery. LDL particles can rapidly penetrate the intact lining of the wall and are trapped in that has been called a "cagework" of fibers there. In this oxygen-rich environment, the LDL is mildly oxidized. Some have compared this reaction to the mild oxidation of butter or margarine left out of refrigeration. This leads to inflammatory changes in the artery wall which do not occur with unoxidized LDL. The tendency to the inflammatory changes is inherited. Oxidized LDL activates certain materials which speed formation of the arterial clots, which can eventually lead to heart attacks and strokes.

The jury is still out on the antioxidant question. The antioxidants usually considered are beta-carotene (which the body converts to vitamin A), vitamin C, and vitamin E. Some of the most important observational studies have been done by a Harvard group, which compared intake of foods containing these substances, as well as vitamin pills, with the incidence of vascular disease. Their Physicians Health Study stopped at the end of 1995 after twelve years, during which administration of beta-carotene on alternate days had neither a beneficial nor a harmful effect in regard to its effect on cancer, the primary end-point for this agent. Earlier it had been rumored that beta-carotene had been associated with reduction in heart attacks, a surprise since the study was intended to measure the effect of alternate-day aspirin on heart attacks and beta-carotene on cancer. Another surprise was that aspirin seemed to reduce colon cancer a little. However, if there appeared to be any beneficial effect on coronary disease from beta-carotene, it must have disappeared in the later years of the study because it was not mentioned at its conclusion.

The Nurses' Health Study, begun by the Harvard group in 1976, was modified in 1980 to include investigation of vitamin E in prevention of CHD. Its intake from food sources and vitamin supplements was compared with reported coronary disease. Subjects with the highest intake of beta-carotene showed a 22% lower risk for CHD than those with the lowest intake; for vitamin E the difference was a 34% reduction in risk. The benefits were seen *only in those who took supplements*; risk was not reduced in those whose intake of vitamin E, however high, was from dietary sources alone. Possibly those who took the supplements were a self-selected group, more attentive to health matters, who smoked less and exercised more. The authors did not believe this could account for this degree of risk reduction, which they attributed to the vitamin.

Harvard's Health Professionals Study evaluated the effects of antioxidant intake in nearly 40,000 various health professionals over four years. Those with highest intake of beta-carotene had a 25% reduction in CHD risk; those with the highest intake of vitamin E had a 39% risk reduction, again only in persons who took *supplemental vitamins*. Increased vitamin C intake provided no significant risk reduction.

When randomized clinical trials are done to test the observations, it sometimes is a different story. In 1995 Jha and associates (Hamilton, Ontario) wrote a critical review of epidemiologic and clinical trial data on antioxidants. They concluded that epidemiologic data suggest that antioxidant vitamins reduce CHD, with the clearest effect for vitamin E; however, *completed randomized trials do not support this finding*. Their final word: Much of this controversy should be resolved by the ongoing large-scale and long-term randomized trials designed specifically to evaluate effects on cardiovascular disease.

As I said, the jury is still out.

Is it true that some drugs increase cholesterol? Does this matter?

Some do, but not by very much and nothing to worry about. The effects of diuretics and beta-blockers are important because many persons with cholesterol problems also are being treated for high blood pressure, and these are the recommended first-line drugs. Diuretics, if they raise TC and LDLC at all, cause mild elevations that don't really matter. If you have been worrying about this, forget it. If a person has a significant cholesterol problem, you treat it with niacin or other appropriate drug; if not, you don't. On the other hand, if you are having trouble raising a low HDLC level and the patients is taking a beta-blocker, you may wish to stop the beta-blocker and observe the HDLC, which can be reduced by that group of agents. I hate to do this since beta-blockers are known to reduce the risk of heart attacks.

What is the effect of alcohol on cholesterol levels?

The best review of this subject was a conference several years ago by three respected experts, Daniel Steinberg (San Diego), Thomas Pearson (Cooperstown, NY) and Lewis Kuller (Pittsburgh). The authors pointed out that epidemiologic data generally show a reduction in CHD risk with moderate alcohol intake (variously defined as two to four drinks a day). However, the potentially drastic effects of excessive alcohol intake on health precludes any recommendation that patients increase their alcohol consumption, The mechanism by which alcohol "protects," if it does, is not clear but may be related to increasing HDLC. Alcohol markedly increases triglyceride-rich lipoproteins and is one of the most common causes of elevated triglycerides. Once liver damage occurs from excessive drinking, HDLC levels may actually be lower than normal.

High alcohol intakes are associated with increased overall mortality. Until we know more about the metabolic and behavioral effects of alcohol and about its linkage to atherosclerosis, we have no basis for recommending either that patients increase their alcohol intake or that they start drinking if they do not already, the authors concluded.

I am not going to talk about red wine having a possible protective effect. When white wine makers developed their own data, they seemed to indicate that white wine had the same possible protective activity. (Remember one of our questions: Who sponsored the study?) Then along came Folts and associates (Madison), who found that drinking six glasses of grape juice daily appears to have the same "anti-clogging" effects as two glasses of red wine. They pointed out that "it's not the alcohol, but the flavonoids"—hundreds of naturally occurring compounds found in the skins, stems, and seeds of grapes—that gives red wine its ability to reduce stickiness of platelets, the little blood cells that stick together and start the clotting process. Thus it would appear that any effect on HDL is not the mechanism of protection by red wine, if there is any. Instead, its value is due to flavonoid-induced reduction in platelet adhesiveness, similar to the action of aspirin, which makes it protective against heart attacks and strokes. Folts does not really advise six glasses of grape juice daily; instead he invites people to follow his example by eating more fresh fruits and vegetables.

What about miscellaneous things to reduce cholesterol— nuts, fish oils, garlic, etc.?

In the long book I discussed these things for a couple of pages. Here I'll just save your time by advising you to save your money and turn your attention to other things such as being good at niacin. These things fall under the heading of Gordon Gould's analogy, throwing something different into the furnace when we should be looking for the thermostat.

I tend to become irritated when anyone wastes time and money on these or other miscellaneous things alleged to affect cholesterol. Using any of these ideas exemplifies a type of weirdness which is all too common in American people today: trying something based on rumors, while not availing themselves of the benefits of current medical knowledge by seeing a doctor. As nearly as I can decipher it, the reasoning must be: the garlic (or other nonsensical regimen) isn't that expensive, it is "natural" [So is strychnine!], and seeing a doctor costs money. This reasoning could cost your life if you really need cholesterol control.

This attitude reminds me of a remark I overheard in an elevator at the Mayo Clinic during my training years there. One passenger said to another, in all seriousness, "Do you believe in doctors?" I still haven't figured that one out. If they didn't, what were they doing there?

Does coffee increase the risk of cardiovascular disease?

No.

Does lipid apheresis have a role in cholesterol control?

Yes, for the unfortunate homozygous [inherited from both parents] familial hypercholesteremic patient doomed to early death from vascular disease (usually heart attack, sometimes in the first decade of life). For such patients who fail to respond to maximal lipid-lowering drug therapy (usually drug combinations) along with dietary change, this can be an important method of treatment. Once or twice a week the patient's blood plasma is run through a machine containing an adsorbent which selectively removes apolipoprotein B, containing LDL and Lp(a), both of which are reduced by this treatment.

196

This investigative treatment may eventually bring a successful long-term approach to persons with homozygous familial hypercholesteremia (FH) as renal dialysis has helped those with chronic renal failure. However, a patient on renal dialysis may be rescued from lifelong dependence on the machine by a kidney transplant. To transplant a liver, which would be necessary in FH and has sometimes been done, is more formidable.

Possibly genetic counseling, attempting to avoid child-bearing in parents who both have the FH gene, will eventually be a more satisfactory answer to this problem.

Could Gene Therapy Control Severe Hypercholesteremia?

Maybe some day.

What is the mechanism of action of niacin?
"How does it work?"

When a new method of treatment is first discovered, its mechanism of action often is not understood. So it was with niacin. From my viewpoint as a practicing internist and clinical investigator, what mattered was that it did everything right. Although curious about what went on in the body to achieve these changes, I was not at a large research facility with the scientists, equipment, and grants to study the mechanism. Some of our early papers speculated about possible mechanisms of action, which we tended to rule out on clinical grounds or admit that, however attractive the theories were, we could not prove them. I repeated speculated that the drug's mode of action might be found by exploring why nicotinic acid (niacin) reduced total cholesterol so dramatically while its close relative, nicotinamide (niacinamide), did not. When Miller and Hamilton (New Orleans) found that the body converts part of niacin to nicotinuric acid, a product not excreted when the amide is administered, it looked as though this might be the key to the drug's action, but it was not. In those days, we wrote like deep thinkers, but actually it was all guesswork.

Eventually there was evidence that niacin inhibited formation by the liver of very low-density lipoprotein (VLDL), from which the body makes LDL. This explains the reduction in LDLC and TC but not the rise in HDLC or reduction in triglycerides. In 1962 Carlson and Oro (Stockholm) first reported that niacin reduces free fatty acids and triglycerides in the blood, apparently by inhibiting breakdown of fat in tissues. They also found that fairly low plasma levels of niacin will reduce cholesterol if they are maintained for a fairly long period of time (hours).

In 1983 Hotz (Frankfurt-Am-Main) published a very thorough review of work pertaining to niacin's mechanism of action. That may seem a long time ago, but there haven't been many basic studies of the mechanism of action in the years since then. Hotz considered the inhibition of fat breakdown into fatty acids to be a more important mechanism than inhibition of VLDL formation. His review did not address the increase in HDLC, and I am not aware of any subsequent work that has. This returns me to my position of knowing *what* niacin does but not being able to explain exactly *how* it accomplishes all its favorable effects.

A story which made the rounds during my training at the Mayo Clinic parallels my longstanding viewpoint on this matter. Recently I verified its authenticity with the principal character. There were four or five Fellows (Rochester term for resident physicians) on the Metabolic Service at St. Mary's Hospital each quarter, with a different consultant on the hospital service each month. One of the consultants, an excellent teacher (as most of them were), would take his group to the cafeteria for coffee in the middle of rounds each morning and pose a provocative question for discussion.

At that time insulin's precise mechanism of action was not known, although it had been used to treat diabetes since its discovery in 1922. The question of the morning was, "What is the mechanism of action of insulin? How does insulin work?" Each of the first few Fellows showed his knowledge of the subject by proposing a complicated theoretical mechanism. Then they came to the last Fellow, Dr. Fred Spencer, a Texan, a little too heavy, who was sitting in the corner of the booth, puffing on a stubby cigar.

The consultant again posed the question: "Dr. Spencer, how do you think insulin works?" Fred puffed his cigar a time or two, then announced to the group, "I think it works just dandy!"

When I am speaking and some one asks me how niacin works, I think of Fred Spencer; in fact, I tell the audience about him. Then I tell them, "I think it works just dandy! It does everything right."

CONCLUSION

What Does All This Mean to the Patient? To the Physician?

Just about everything good in the practice of medicine is accomplished by a team, the patient and the physician, both knowledgeable in what they are trying to achieve and how to reach the goals. The information in this book can impart the needed knowledge. The patient and physician must now use it together.

Reminders for Both Patient and Physician

Both of you should know that diet is not necessary to control cholesterol. Diet must be used only if weight control is also an issue, in which case there is no substitute for calorie control. There is an urgent need to combat the epidemic of obesity in this country. The large percentage of our population who are overweight or outright obese are people sacrificing quality of life in younger years by not looking and feeling good; at the same time they are wearing out their weight-bearing joints, which will further ruin the quality of life in later years.

Patient and physician should remember always that niacin has so many advantages, not shared by any other drugs for cholesterol control, that it is truly a designer drug. *It is highly unlikely that another drug will ever come along which has all of these distinctive advantages.* Remember that niacin:

1) Reduces total cholesterol (TC) and LDL ("bad") cholesterol (LDLC)

2) Increases HDL ("good") cholesterol (HDLC)

3) Reduces triglycerides

4) Lessens the likelihood of heart attack, stroke and related events, cardiovascular surgery, cardiovascular hospitalization, and all hospitalization

199

5) Reduces Lp(a), as does no other treatment, except estrogens in postmenopausal women

6) Favorably alters subfractions of HDLC

7) Favorably alters particle size in subfractions of LDLC

8) Attains all these goals at a cost about one-sixth to one-tenth that of the largest-selling cholesterol-control drugs, the statins

9) Accomplishes all the above-listed goals while the patient eats an ordinary American diet

All these actions are important, but the last statement is worth emphasizing for those who think they must live on a low-fat, egg-free, highly fibrous diet they neither want nor need. *You don't have to diet to control cholesterol!* We included this good news in nearly all of the early publications on the success of what we then called nicotinic acid in the late 1950's and early 1960's. It still holds true today.

Both patient and physician should remember that all these distinctive advantages will *not* be widely publicized, unless through this book, if it should achieve widespread recognition. As long as niacin remains generic and inexpensive, no manufacturer realizes enough profits even to consider trying to compete with the media blitzes of the big-spending producers of expensive cholesterol-control drugs. Diet advocates and niacin detractors will do everything they can to divert attention from the truths listed here. They include the companies producing other drugs for cholesterol control, whose actions do not begin to match the benefits just listed for niacin, and the food industry, with its huge advertising budgets.

In certain instances, when the body factory's defect in producing cholesterol appears to be mild and is limited to elevated LDLC, the patient and physician might want to try a dietary approach to the cholesterol abnormality. In that case, they should realize that if the goals of treatment have not been achieved and are not being approached *in two months*, they should proceed to drug therapy. Before considering such a trial, the physician should be sure that the patient knows two important facts:

1) The diet you are going to follow for those two months must be the diet you are willing to follow daily for the rest of your life.

2) You don't have to diet to control cholesterol!

Both patient and physician should know that eggs in the diet have little or nothing to do with the level of cholesterol in the blood. If there still exists a doubt, review the discussion earlier in the book (Chapter 4). If the doctor is uncertain about whether a patient might be "egg-sensitive," an "egg test" is simple to do. As you recall, this consists of checking cholesterol levels on the present program (usually few or no eggs), then eating all the eggs one desires for a month and rechecking the levels.

The cost factor is worth re-emphasizing. Just compare niacin's cost, about $8 to $10 a month, to that of the largest-selling drugs (statins) at $55 to more than $200 per month. Even using $120 a year as the cost of niacin, Mevacor, priced at $55 a month for its starting dose, 20 mg a day, comes to $660 a year, 5.5 times as much. Prices for the new, trendy Lipitor are similar for the lowest dose($55 a month) but even higher ($222 a month) if the maximum recommended dose, 80 mg, were ever used. Those who like to think about large numbers can project this to the millions of Americans who are candidates for cholesterol control by current NCEP guidelines. If most of them (possibly as many as 90%, if all doctors were good at niacin) could take this inexpensive designer drug instead of statins, the savings would be billions of dollars annually. These figures should be of vital interest to government and to managed care organizations, both of whom should support wide distribution of this book.

But as you know by now, I think in terms of the individual approach to such matters. To me, the difference is $540 in your pocket every year, the difference between $120 (niacin) and $660 (Mevacor, Lipitor).

To The Patient

To receive the benefits of cholesterol control by niacin, the patient must take certain responsibilities. First, learn what your cholesterol levels are: total cholesterol (TC), LDL cholesterol (LDLC), and HDL cholesterol (HDLC). See how they compare with my version of the current NCEP guidelines:

1) HDLC 45 or above in everyone

2) LDLC below 100 if any previous cardiovascular event (heart attack, anginal pain, coronary artery bypass surgery/angioplasty/ atherectomy/stent; stroke or related event, leg pains due to im- paired circulation, surgery on neck arteries or leg arteries

3) LDLC below 130 in everyone else with two or more risk factors from this list:

- Male sex or postmenopausal female
- Current smoker

- High blood pressure
- Diabetes
- Inadequate physical exercise
- Obesity (more than 30% above ideal weight)
- HDLC below 35
- Family history of any above-listed cardiovascular event, or sudden death, before age 55 in first-degree[1] male relative or before age 65 in first-degree female relative

4) LDLC below 160 in those who do not have two or more risk factors, as just listed

Most middle-aged adults will have two or more risk factors from the above list since male sex or postmenopausal female will automatically give them one. Only among young adults are we likely to find persons who fall into the last category with fewer than two risk factors. That's why I say "LDL less than 130 for nearly everyone."

If your cholesterol fractions are all within desirable levels, you need do nothing more except have the levels checked periodically. In young adults, this can be about every three years. In persons over 40, an annual examination is desirable; this includes blood tests which always include TC. Be sure your doctor specifies at least HDLC as well. From this the LDLC can be calculated, even if you are not fasting, using a mathematical trick I shall spell out for doctors in the next section.

If you have had an event, as defined in item 2, above, NCEP guidelines call it imperative to bring your LDLC level below 100. I agree. This almost always requires drug therapy, so niacin should be foremost in your thoughts and those of your physician. If you have not had an event and are over 70, discuss with your doctor whether your pattern of cholesterol fractions should be treated, in view of any other medical conditions. If you are a woman, be sure your doctor treats your lipid levels to those listed above. Do not take no for an answer. Do not let the physician hide behind the ACP naysayer guidelines, which basically excluded everyone from treatment except middle-aged men with known coronary disease. We reviewed these foolish guidelines in the Medical Section (*A View Disagreeing with NCEP Recommendations*).

---

[1] A first-degree relative is a parent, sibling, or offspring.

If you are a young adult, you may be your own worst enemy if you fail to follow the NCEP guidelines. We can learn an important lesson from the tragic story of Sergei Grinkov, the 28-year-old Russian figure skater whose sudden death shocked the world late in 1995. In superb condition, he had just rehearsed a program with his wife, his skating partner, when he complained of dizziness and slumped to the ice, dead of a heart attack. There had been warnings for anyone who noticed them. Four years earlier his father had died suddenly at 52 after three previous heart attacks. Sergei was known to have high blood pressure (treated, I would hope). In press reports I saw, nothing was ever said about his cholesterol level or fractions, leading me to believe these had not been examined carefully, as they should have been in a young man with these risk factors. Autopsy revealed that he had blockage of two coronary arteries and had suffered a heart attack 24 hours before his death. Apparently it was a silent heart attack; otherwise, he had either a high pain threshold or a lot of disease denial.

Young adults should have cholesterol fractions measured and other risk factors assessed on the same basis as older adults. Of all age groups, young persons have the most to gain by discovering abnormal risk factors early and treating them properly.

It is important for patients—not just you, who are already reading it, but every patient—to buy and read this book. After reading it, keep it for future reference. Some day you may want to refresh your memory about some of the fine points or rare problems before talking to your doctor about them. Always remember the primary lesson this book teaches: *Niacin is not a do-it-yourself drug. Its use requires knowledgeable medical supervision.*

Except for diabetics who require insulin, anyone who has read the book and realizes he is a candidate for cholesterol control should *buy another copy of the book and give it to his doctor.* As Chapter 9 suggested, tell him you want him to be *good at niacin,* and with the book he can accomplish this in a few evenings of reading. Then remind yourself of my advice on what to do if your physician rejects out of hand the idea that he become good at niacin and possibly use it for you. ("My best advice is simple: *change doctors!* Change doctors? *Of course. Your life is at stake.*") Having read this book, you will know how to find a doctor who is good at niacin or is willing to get there with this simple guide.

The patient must be willing to work with the doctor, using this book as her guide. When you are taking niacin, accept your responsibility to have your cholesterol levels measured and see the doctor at the stated intervals—

monthly during periods of dosage adjustment, 12-week intervals when things are going smoothly and all fractions are on target.

Never be backward about discussing your niacin therapy with your physician. Based on your reading this book, you may have valid information he has missed or forgotten, even though he did read the book. By bringing up a question or discussing a fine point, you may help not only yourself but others as well.

To the Physician

Having read the book to this point, you should now be good at niacin. What final thoughts should I leave with you? When we finish this section, please let me know whether you think I have placed the emphasis properly.

In my opinion, any doctor who realizes niacin's distinctive advantages in lipid control and the tremendous cost difference between it and less effective drugs will make niacin his personal drug of choice. If you are good at niacin, more than 90% of your patients who need lipid control will be able to take the drug successfully and, almost without exception, to achieve the goals of treatment. How much your percentage exceeds 90% will depend on how adept you become in its use.

If you were not already aware, having been brainwashed by the media, opinion-making bodies, and representatives of expensive drugs, you will soon begin to find out that the alleged disadvantages of niacin practically all disappear into thin air when you use the drug skillfully. The flush, *much over-rated* in the first place and over-inflated by niacin detractors, is seldom a problem if you use aspirin each morning and prescribe TRNA as your starting drug. My recommended 1-2-3 dosage schedule over the first few weeks will usually be well tolerated and will identify the few persons who develop nausea at these modest doses. Nausea can usually be sorted out by stopping the drug for a week or two, then resuming it to see whether the symptom recurs.

When using plain niacin, I now use Endurance Products Plain Niacin (EP NA), with its dissolution time of about 50 minutes. I prefer it to the old-fashioned unmodified niacin (NA), which dissolves in three to five minutes, with a correspondingly rapid occurrence of flushing—at least at first. My current plan reserves EP NA for persons who have nausea or significant alteration of liver function tests (enzyme levels more than twice normal) when they take TRNA, or for those who need greater increases in HDLC than TRNA achieves. In the latter situation, one can replace part or all of the TRNA with EP NA. If nausea or liver function abnormalities are the reason for the change, I stop TRNA and replace it entirely with EP NA. At first I wondered whether EP NA might, like the earlier intermediate-release product, aluminum nicotinate (Nicalex), have a profile for nausea and liver function abnormalities midway between unmodified NA and TRNA. To date this has not happened in two years of use. However, it appears that EP NA might be more effective in lower doses than the old, unmodified NA tablets.

Let me give you my mathematical trick for estimating LDLC if the patient was not fasting or if your laboratory has done only TC and HDLC. *Add 20 to the HDLC.* (In most people, VDLC will be between 15 and 25, so I use 20 as an arbitrary figure.) Since TC = HDLC + VLDLC + LDLC, *subtract this number (HDLC + 20) from TC.* The result will be very close to the correct LDLC level.

This trick works whether the serum sample is fasting or after eating. Compare it to your laboratory's calculation of LDLC by the Friedewald equation (valid only if the patient has been fasting, because only then will the triglycerides, which enter into the calculation, be accurate). See how close it usually comes. You may also want to look at the VLDL level when you obtain a lipid profile, noticing the occasional patient who has a VLDLC higher that the usual 15 to 25 range. However, when using niacin, VLDLC is usually reduced to a normal level if it has been high.

Find out the costs of a lipid profile (TC, LDLC, HDLC, VLDLC, triglycerides) in your laboratory and compare it to the charge for just TC and HDLC. In our setting, it has sometimes cost a little less for the entire profile. Of course, the full profile should be done on fasting blood, as noted above. In a nonfasting sample, I use my mathematical trick to calculate the LDLC.

I hope physicians who read this book will avoid all the common errors in cholesterol management with niacin:

◆ The worst error, I suppose, would be to *ignore cholesterol entirely*; next to that would be to look just at TC without considering the fractions. *Total cholesterol is really irrelevant if both LDLC and HDLC are in desirable ranges.*

◆ The second common error is *to think a "cholesterol-lowering" diet will be effective,* sentencing a patient to this approach, and *not checking in two months* to see whether the goals of treatment are being achieved or at least approached. Remember, most persons will not follow a diet strict enough to control the output of the body's cholesterol factory; even if they do, diet more often than not is ineffective in reaching the goals.

◆ Another attitude in some doctors not good at niacin is *not to treat women, young persons, or elderly persons* with cholesterol patterns outside the current guidelines. I hope our discussion of these situations in the Medical Section will eliminate such omissions. The best way to make a doctor more aware of who needs cholesterol control is to make him good at niacin. When you know exactly how handle problems with cholesterol fractions (and at low cost to the patient), you are more likely to use your skills for more people who deserve to be treated.

◆ As we have said repeatedly, failing to select niacin as your first-choice drug would be a mistake. Let's hope this book will eliminate that error.

◆ Probably the *most common* error in prescribing niacin is to follow the prevalent advice in modern literature, which says *to start plain niacin with a low dose and increase it gradually.* For plain niacin, 1000 mg three times a day from the start makes the flush subside earlier and saves all that wasted time in reaching an effective dose. For TRNA, I have already repeated my first-month plan (third paragraph of *To the Physician*, the 1-2-3 plan). For EP Plain Niacin, I feel that a dose a little lower than that for unmodified niacin is probably advisable. Its very existence and widespread use could revolutionize therapy with plain niacin since EP NA virtually eliminates flushing and makes it unnecessary even to think of starting at a low dose.

◆ Although the "low and slow" error may be the most common, at least it only wastes time. The *most serious error* by a doctor not good at niacin is to *find a minor increase in one or more liver function tests and stop the drug,* fearing that this means hepatic toxicity. He needs to know that such minor elevations are *a normal part* of niacin therapy in some persons, are not progressive, and do not require a change in dosage. For example, a doctor may see SGOT and SGPT levels of, let's say, 61 to 75 (normals 41 to 45). The proper action is to continue the program if lipid levels are satisfactory and the patient is free of symptoms. The inexperienced doctor may panic and abandon niacin, perhaps forever, thus denying his patient its benefits. Of course, if transaminase levels rise to *two to three times the upper limit of normal,* it is well to stop the drug and consider another option after the abnormal levels return to normal, usually within two weeks. If TRNA caused the changes, the option might be to use NA or EP NA. With these products the goals may be reached without nausea or significant changes in liver tests.

◆ Another possible error would be *to worry about the slight increases in glucose or uric acid,* or, even worse, stop niacin for either of these reasons.

206

The same comment applies to *skin dryness* or the *skin changes resembling acanthosis nigricans.*

Having become good at niacin, what can you, the physician, do to bring its benefits to all your patients who need it? (Remember, this includes at least 29% of American adults.) You may find this book useful in teaching your patients to understand and use the drug.

What else can you do to bring its benefits to others, beyond your own practice? Here is a partial list. You may think of others.

◆ Become evangelistic. Recommend the book and the use of niacin to your medical colleagues.

◆ Do the same for your pharmacists, so they too will become good at niacin, instead of misleading patients, as some have done by not knowing the important differences between NA and TRNA.

◆ Encourage your pharmacies to stock Endur-acin, EP NA, and Slo-Niacin. The manufacturer of Endur-acin and EP Plain Niacin has assured me that the company could meet the demand for these products if other pharmacies (in addition to Walgreen's and some independent pharmacies, who now have them) wanted to sell them. Expanded availability of these products in pharmacies would be desirable. Patients, who must remember to stay under the doctor's supervision, might want to consider ordering the products directly from the company. This gives them more options regarding bottle sizes since the stores, so far at least, only carry bottles of 100 caplets.[2]

◆ Take the book's message to your local American Heart Association affiliate. Try to get them to understand that the AHA's antiquated stance is wrong. Tell them you and your patients are tired of hearing it. You *don't* have to diet to control cholesterol!—if your doctor is good at niacin.

◆ Use your own stature and credibility in your community to convince your local news media that the book's message is valid. Get the media to tell patients about the information the book contains for them, including my instructions to patients in this chapter.

◆ Participate in saving billions of dollars annually by leading the change from expensive drugs to niacin, one patient at a time.

---

[2] To order supplies from Endurance Products Company, Tigard, Oregon, one can call the 800 number on each bottle of Endur-acin (1-800-547-1884). The company tells me that orders received in the morning go out that afternoon, postage paid. In addition to the bottles of 100 sold in pharmacies, patients may order bottles of 600 or 1000.

◆ Bring the cost-effectiveness of niacin therapy to the attention of your hospital pharmacy and of managed-care organizations, emphasizing that each doctor must be good at niacin for these economies to be realized.

◆ Let the National Cholesterol Education Program (NCEP) at National Institutes of Health (NIH) know that you would like the truths of this book spelled out in their next set of guidelines—which would require at least one niacin-knowledgeable member on the "Expert Panel." Until now there have been none.

◆ Tell drug sales representatives (or the companies directly) the shortcomings of their expensive drugs for cholesterol control. Tell them you are tired of having them spend multi-millions on advertising their drugs and on clinical trials for which the unsuspecting public pays.

◆ Let the food industry know you are tired of their big-budget advertising, based on implied benefits of "low-fat" or "low-cholesterol" foods, which are not needed to control cholesterol and usually are not effective. Tell them to quit exhorting the American public to follow a low-fat, low-cholesterol, no-egg, fibrous diet they neither want nor need.

◆ Let me know what you are doing to make a difference in any of the above ways, or in ways you may think of but which I have not listed.

Does this sound like a crusade? It should be. Joseph Poindexter, a Senior Editor of *People* magazine, called my work with niacin "a lonely odyssey." I hope it will no longer be lonely.

I would like my earlier statement about hope for the future to be the closing benediction: "The food industry will survive. Its managers will change their 'low cholesterol' marketing strategy to 'low in calories' or even 'good to eat' ads when it becomes widely known that low-fat, low-cholesterol diets are not necessary, often not effective, and perhaps not even safe. The winners will be the people of the world, whose lives and dinner-table conversation will no longer center on the effect they believe each bite might have on their serum cholesterol levels and their arteries. Perhaps we can get back to basics: eat food because it tastes good, exercise because it feels good, control weight because it looks good, and be happy—because life should be enjoyed, one day at a time."

Definitions of Medical Terms and Abbreviations Used in This Book

Acanthosis nigricans—a skin disorder characterized by patches of velvety tan to brown pigmentation in localized areas

Albumin—the most abundant protein in blood serum, formed in the liver

Alpha$_1$-lipoprotein cholesterol—an old term (1950's, 1960's) for what we now call high-density lipoprotein (HDL) cholesterol; "good" cholesterol

ALT—alanine aminotransferase, an enzyme produced only in the liver, measurable in blood, used as a test of liver function; same as SGPT

AMA—American Medical Association, usually [As the story goes, the president of the American Motorcycle Association once wrote to the president of the American Medical Association, "It has come to my attention that you are using the initials of our organization..."]

AMWA—American Medical Women's Association

Angina pectoris, angina—pain or discomfort in the chest, or sometimes other areas, caused by insufficient blood flow to heart muscle through the coronary arteries

Anticoagulant—a drug administered to lessen the ability of the blood to clot

Arteriography—imaging of arteries by x-ray, using injections of materials into the arteries

AST—aspartate aminotransferase, an enzyme product produced in the liver and other tissues, measurable in blood, used as a test of liver function in conjunction with other tests; same as SGOT

Atherosclerosis—narrowing of arteries by plaques within their inner walls, composed of cholesterol and other materials

Atorvastatin—generic name for Lipitor, a drug used for cholesterol and triglyceride control

Atromid-S—trade name for clofibrate, a lipid-altering drug studied in the Coronary Drug Project but now seldom used in the U.S.

"Bad" cholesterol—low-density lipoprotein (LDL) cholesterol

Beta-blockers—drugs used to treat high blood pressure and heart disease, which act by blocking the effect of adrenalin (produced by the body) on heart and blood vessels

Beta-lipoprotein cholesterol—an old term (1950's, 1960's) for low-density lipoprotein (LDL) cholesterol; "bad" cholesterol

Bile acid sequestrant—a material (resin) which attaches itself to bile acids in the intestine and carries them out of the body, making them unavailable for reabsorption and further formation of cholesterol

Cardiovascular—pertaining to the heart and blood vessels

CDP—Coronary Drug Project, an important study of lipid-altering drugs and heart disease (1966-1974)

Cholesterol—the most important lipid (fat-like substance) in the blood because of its role in formation of deposits in the walls of arteries, leading to heart attacks, strokes, or other impairment of arterial blood supply

Cholesterol fractions—low-density lipoprotein cholesterol (LDLC), high-density lipoprotein cholesterol (HDLC), and very low density lipoprotein cholesterol (VLDLC)

Cholestyramine—generic name for a bile-sequestrant resin (trade name Questran), administered for cholesterol reduction

Choloxin—trade name for d-thyroxine, a thyroid-like compound formerly used for cholesterol reduction, abandoned after its poor showing in the Coronary Drug Project

Claudication—discomfort, usually pain, in muscles, usually in the legs, functioning with an inadequate supply of blood, often referred to as "intermittent claudication" because it occurs with exercise, subsides with rest, but recurs with more exercise

Clofibrate—a fibric acid derivative (trade name Atromid-S), formerly used in the U.S. and in the Coronary Drug Project, now replaced in U.S. by gemfibrozil

Coagulation—clotting, usually referring to blood

Colestid—trade name for colestipol, a bile-sequestrant resin for cholesterol reduction

Colestipol—generic name for that resin

Coronary artery—one of the system of arteries which run on the surface of the heart (like a crown—Latin, corona), furnishing the blood supply to heart muscle

Coronary Drug Project—a landmark study of lipid-altering drugs and cardiovascular disease (1966-1974)

CPK—creatine phosphokinase, an enzyme in heart muscle and skeletal muscle, released into the blood stream in damage to either type of muscle

CT scan, CAT scan—computerized axial tomography, a method of imaging portions of the body (head, chest, abdomen) by "slices," showing the relationship of solid organs to one another

Cutaneous—referring to the skin

Diabetes mellitus—the inherited disorder in carbohydrate metabolism commonly called "diabetes"

Dilatation—widening or enlarging, as in blood vessels, or pupils of the eyes

d-thyroxine—a thyroid-like compound (trade name Choloxin) once used for cholesterol reduction

Double-blind study—an experiment in which neither the participant nor the investigator knows who is receiving an active drug and who is receiving a placebo; any similar experiment

-emia—a suffix referring to blood; e.g., anemia (lack of blood); hypercholesteremia (high blood cholesterol); hyperglycemia (high blood glucose)

Endur-acin—a time-release niacin preparation (Endurance Products, Tigard, Oregon), used for cholesterol control

EP Plain Niacin—a product of Endurance Products which dissolves in just less than an hour (hence, Plain), introduced in 1996, used for cholesterol control

Fluvastatin—generic name for Lescol, a drug used for cholesterol control

Foam cell—a macrophage (scavenger cell of the body) laden with lipids, which enters the wall of an artery and participates in the formation of an atherosclerotic plaque

Framingham Study—a study lasting more than a quarter of a century (in Framingham, Massachusetts), which developed more information regarding coronary risk factors than any other in history

Gemfibrozil—a fibric acid derivative (trade name Lopid), used for treatment of certain lipid abnormalities

GGTP, or GGT—gamma-glutamyltransferase, an enzyme produced in liver, measurable in blood, used as a test of liver function

Globulins—a group of serum proteins produced in the liver

Glucose—a sugar normally present in blood

Glycosuria—glucose in the urine, an abnormal finding usually signifying diabetes

"Good" cholesterol—high density lipoprotein cholesterol (HDLC)

HDL, or HDLC—high density lipoprotein, or high density lipoprotein cholesterol; "good" cholesterol

HDL$_2$, HDL$_3$—two subfractions of "good" cholesterol (HDLC)

Hepatic—referring to the liver; e.g., hepatic function tests, hepatic toxicity

Hyper—a prefix denoting too high or too much

Hypercholesteremia, hypercholesterolemia—high blood cholesterol [I prefer the shorter spelling.]

Hyperglycemia—high blood sugar

Hyperlipidemia—high levels of lipids (fat-like substances) in blood; usually refers to cholesterol and/or triglycerides

Hypertension—high blood pressure [Does *not* refer to excess nervous tension.]

Hyperthyroidism—excessive activity of the thyroid gland

Hyperuricemia—elevated levels of uric acid in blood

Hypo—a prefix denoting too low or too little

Hypoglycemia—lower than normal levels of glucose in the blood

Hypothyroidism—reduced or insufficient activity of the thyroid gland

Infarction—damage to tissue deprived of its oxygen-carrying blood supply

Insulin—a protein hormone, made by the pancreas, which controls glucose metabolism

Ischemia—lack or insufficiency of blood flow

LDL, or LDLC—low density lipoprotein or low density lipoprotein cholesterol; "bad" cholesterol

Lescol—trade name for fluvastatin, a drug for cholesterol control

Lipid—a fat-like substance; in this book usually refers to cholesterol and/or triglycerides

Lipid profile—a group of blood tests to evaluate a person's status regarding cholesterol, its fractions, and triglycerides

Lipitor—trade name for atorvastatin, a drug used for cholesterol and triglyceride control

Lipoprotein—a compound with a protein base carrying varying amounts and types of lipids (cholesterol and triglycerides)

Lopid—trade name for gemfibrozil, a drug used to treat certain lipid abnormalities

Lorelco—trade name for probucol, a drug formerly used for cholesterol control

Lovastatin—generic name for Mevacor, a drug used for cholesterol control

Lp(a)—abbreviation for lipoprotein (a), a variant of LDL cholesterol which is a predictor of risk of coronary disease

LRCT—Lipid Research Clinics Trial (my shortening from a longer title), a study of resin (cholestyramine), cholesterol reduction, and cardiovascular disease

Lumen—the space within a tubular organ, such as a blood vessel or intestine

Macrophage—a cell which acts as a sort of scavenger in body tissues; when laden with lipids, it becomes a "foam cell," which participates in formation of the atherosclerotic plaque in the arterial wall

Mean (as in *mean* cholesterol levels)—for all practical purposes, may be read as "average" levels

Mevacor—trade name for lovastatin, a drug used for cholesterol control

Myalgia—pain in muscles

Myopathy—literally, something wrong in muscle(s)

Myositis—inflammation in muscle(s)

Myocardial infarction—heart attack, with damage to heart muscle due to lack of adequate blood supply

Myocardium—heart muscle

NA—nicotinic acid, niacin (used in this book to abbreviate *plain niacin)*

NCEP—National Cholesterol Education Program, an activity of NIH

NHLBI—National Heart, Lung, and Blood Institute, part of NIH (at one time just National Heart Institute)

NIA—National Institute on Aging

Niacin—a member of the vitamin B complex; used in large doses to control cholesterol, it is a drug, not a vitamin

Niacinamide—closely related to niacin, has vitamin activity but does not affect cholesterol

Nicotinamide—same as niacinamide

Nicotinic acid—same as niacin

NIH—National Institutes of Health (Bethesda, Maryland)

Placebo—an inactive pill, sometimes used in double-blind studies to compare with effects of active drugs

Plaque—a deposit of lipids and other substances within the inner wall of an artery; the basic lesion of atherosclerosis, which narrows arteries and can lead to their blockage

Pravachol—trade name for pravastatin, a drug used for cholesterol control

Premarin—trade name for conjugated equine estrogens, the most frequently used female hormone for menopausal symptoms or lessening of osteoporosis

Probucol—generic name for Lorelco, a drug formerly used for cholesterol control

Prostaglandins—a group of hormone-like substances formed in the body, which have various important functions, including inflammatory changes, reproduction, and other actions, including the cutaneous flush characteristic of niacin use

Questran—trade name for cholestyramine, a bile-sequestrant resin used for cholesterol reduction

Randomized study—one in which participants are assigned to one program or another impartially, by a table of random numbers

Regression studies—trials which have shown that aggressive cholesterol control can result, not only in retardation of new deposits, but in lessening of existing plaques in arteries when studied by arteriography

Renal—referring to the kidneys

Resins—powders whose particles adsorb bile acids, removing them from the body via the intestine

Risk factors—measurable influences which, if beyond a certain range, increase the risk of disease; e.g., smoking, high blood pressure, and hypercholesteremia are risk factors for coronary disease

RSS—Really Stupid Studies

SGOT—glutamic oxalacetic transaminase, an enzyme produced in the liver and other tissues, measurable in the blood, used as a liver function test; same as AST

SGPT—glutamic pyruvate transaminase, an enzyme produced only in liver, measurable in blood, used as a liver function test; same as ALT

Simvastatin—generic name for Zocor, a drug used for cholesterol control

Slo-Niacin—a time-release niacin preparation (Upsher-Smith, Minneapolis, Minnesota), used for cholesterol control

Stenosis—narrowing, as in a blood vessel or heart valve

Stent—a device placed within an artery [or in another hollow tube, such as bile duct or ureter] to hold it open, in an effort to prevent blockage

Stroke—an episode in which brain is damaged because of interrupted blood flow by a clot or by a hemorrhage from a broken blood vessel; called a "brain attack" by some authors in recent years

TRNA—time-release nicotinic acid (time-release niacin)

Thyroxine—thyroid hormone

Uric acid—one of the end-products of protein metabolism, measurable in blood, deposited as crystals in joints (gouty arthritis) or kidneys (stones)

VLDL—very low density lipoprotein, from which the body manufactures LDL

VLDLC—very low density lipoprotein cholesterol, the cholesterol component of the above lipoprotein

Zocor—trade name for simvastatin, a drug used for cholesterol control

216

Treatment of Abnormal Blood Cholesterol Levels with Niacin

History

Niacin was originally known as a member of the vitamin B complex. Until 1955 it had no known use in medicine except as a vitamin. In that year three Canadian doctors reported a brief trial in which large doses of niacin reduced blood cholesterol levels. Their idea reached the Mayo Clinic, where a young resident physician (William B. Parsons Jr., M.D.) performed the first systematic study of niacin's cholesterol-lowering effect. He and Mayo colleagues published their report in the spring of 1956. He then continued his studies in Madison, Wisconsin. In the next few years, further studies there, at the Mayo Clinic, and at many centers around the world developed much of our present understanding of niacin's use. One important fact was that niacin controlled cholesterol in the presence of an ordinary American diet. *You don't have to diet to control cholesterol!*

This work led to inclusion of niacin in the Coronary Drug Project (CDP), a nationwide study of cholesterol-altering drugs and heart disease, in 7,700 men who had already had one or more heart attacks. From 1966 to 1974, investigators at 53 centers worked together on this first-ever nationwide cooperative study. Of several drugs in the study, only niacin reduced the rates of heart attacks, strokes and stroke-related events, cardiovascular surgery, cardiovascular hospitalization, and all hospitalization. None of the other drugs (no longer used today) had any of these favorable effects. There was no dietary restriction in the CDP.

Ten years later a follow-up survey showed that only niacin had reduced the over-all death rate of CDP participants. Thus niacin was not only the first effective cholesterol-reducing drug but also the first drug clearly shown to reduce the serious heart and blood vessel complications of atherosclerosis (narrowing of the arteries by cholesterol plaques). Since then, studies have shown that niacin, combined with other drugs, can cause deposits in arteries to regress, as shown by repeated coronary artery x-rays.

Treatment of Hypercholesteremia (High Blood Cholesterol Levels)

In 1988 an "Expert Panel" from the National Cholesterol Education Program (NCEP) of National Institutes of Health (NIH) made recommendations for discovery and treatment of elevated cholesterol levels, which it later revised in 1993. In both reports this group designated *niacin* and *resins* (cholestyramine, or Questran, and colestipol, or Colestid) as "first-line drugs" in treatment of blood cholesterol levels, based on their long safety records and proven ability to reduce not only cholesterol levels but also heart attacks and deaths. In the 1993 guidelines, they changed the designation to "major drugs" and added another group, *coenzyme A reductase inhibitors,* nicknamed "*statins*" since their names end with this suffix.

The NCEP Panel stated that cholesterol levels above 240 clearly needed treatment. Levels below 200 were considered desirable, as even borderline levels between 200 and 240 were associated with an undesirable rate of heart attacks and strokes.

Dietary Treatment

The Expert Panel originally recommended dietary management as a first step in treating cholesterol levels, perhaps for as long as six months. Actually the main factor in determining your blood cholesterol level is what your body factory is doing, *not* what you eat. A 1993 book, *Coronary Heart Disease: The Dietary Sense and Nonsense*, comments further on this point and takes the position that diet does not reduce cholesterol levels except during periods of weight reduction, after which cholesterol rises again.

It would be wrong to say that diet *never* helps cholesterol levels. However, it is correct to say that diet is a *weak and often ineffective method* of controlling cholesterol. Many people have read about dietary measures and are already doing a good job of limiting animal fats in their diets. It is really not necessary to spend six months to see whether diet will control a cholesterol problem. The important question is not what a few months of dietary good behavior will accomplish; it is what diet each person is willing to follow for the rest of his/her life. Since the ultimate question is whether any program brings both bad and good cholesterol fractions to desirable levels, I find that the most acceptable program for most persons is to use niacin in the presence of a normal diet if weight is satisfactory, or to reduce calories significantly if weight is excessive.

Use of Niacin for Hypercholesteremia

Flushing of the Skin from Niacin

Long before its use for cholesterol reduction, niacin had been known to cause flushing of the skin, accompanied by a warm feeling in the face, neck, and upper half of the body, occasionally all over. This occurs when plain niacin is first taken, even in doses as small as 50 mg; it is no more severe when doses of 1000 mg or more are used. In fact, as the Canadians pointed out and Parsons confirmed, taking 1000 mg three times a day resulted in disappearance of the flush early in treatment, averaging three to four days. The time varies in different persons. With plain niacin, flushing occurs right away and lasts perhaps half an hour at first. It is worst the first day and diminishes soon thereafter in most persons. The flush is sometimes accompanied by itching and occasionally by a slightly bumpy rash, both of which should subside as the flush does.

These remarks so far apply to old-fashioned *plain* (or unmodified) niacin. *Time-release* niacin preparations allow the medication to absorb gradually as the tablet or capsule goes through the digestive tract. This greatly reduces the flushing. Some persons have none at all, but most experience a little warmth and perhaps some tingling at one time or another, often several hours after swallowing the drug. There is also a *modified plain* niacin preparation which dissolves in about 50 minutes (compared to 3 to 5 minutes for unmodified plain niacin and 7 to 9 hours for the best time-release product). Another way to reduce or eliminate the flush is to take a regular aspirin tablet (325 mg) first thing in the morning, with 6 to 8 ounces of water. With these several ways to lessen flushing, this should really never become a reason that a patient cannot take niacin.

There are a fair number of time-release niacin products on the market. Since niacin has long been a generic drug, no company holds a patent; any company may produce it. As a result, niacin is quite inexpensive, compared to the recently developed and heavily promoted expensive drugs for cholesterol control. Each time-release product has different absorption characteristics. It is impossible for any doctor to be familiar with all products. Each doctor is wise to become familiar with one or two products and insist that his patients use only those.

> The product I want you to take is: _____
>
> Size of tablet/capsule: _500_ mg
>
> This is a _____ plain _____ time-release niacin product.
>
> Your starting dose should be _____
>
> At the end of the first month, your dose will be _____

Niacin is usually taken with meals. Eat part of your meal, take your tablets, and then finish the meal. This lessens the flush with plain niacin and makes both types absorb better. Many people find that they do not need to take time-release niacin with meals after a while; any time of day or night is all right. It is best to divide the daily amount into two or three doses; taking it all at once is not as effective. If flushing should be a problem, avoiding hot beverages and soups is wise for the first week or so.

Time-release niacin tends to cause more nausea and more change in liver function tests than plain niacin, especially in larger doses. At times it may be desirable to change from time-release niacin to plain niacin, for reasons a knowledgeable physician will know. After the body becomes accustomed to taking niacin in time-release form, a patient can usually switch to plain niacin without flushing.

It is important that a patient not change his niacin preparation (especially from plain niacin to time-release niacin) without his doctor's knowledge and approval. One must read labels carefully to be sure he does not make such a change without realizing it. Changing from plain niacin to time-release niacin in the same mg dose would be a very serious mistake, with extremely serious consequences.

Nausea

Nausea, with or without vomiting, can be a side effect of niacin in a small percentage of patients. If a person experiences nausea, we usually stop niacin for a week or two, then resume its use. If something else caused the nausea, there should be no further problem. If niacin was responsible, nausea will probably recur, in which case it can be eliminated by using a smaller dose or by changing from time-release to plain niacin. Sometimes it is necessary to consider a different drug for cholesterol control. We hope this will not be necessary since niacin has several advantages which none of the other drugs has.

Changes in Liver Function Tests

Several blood enzymes used as liver function tests may be slightly elevated during niacin treatment. By studying the situation carefully in the early 1960's, Parsons found that this slight alteration does not represent actual liver damage. The CDP, in which more than 1,000 men took niacin for five to eight years, found no liver damage associated with niacin or any of the other study drugs. One proof that the mild chemical alterations are not really associated with liver damage is that they return to normal soon after stopping niacin.

However, if the abnormal values rise to two to three times normal, liver damage may be imminent and niacin must be stopped. A doctor skilled in use of niacin knows that even these changes return to normal soon after stopping the drug.

In more than 40 years of niacin's use for cholesterol reduction, there have been two serious instances of liver damage reported, both in the late 1980's. One patient had severe liver damage after changing from a fairly high dose of plain niacin to an equal dose of time-release niacin, which is about the same as doubling the dose. In less than a week he was seriously ill with liver damage and survived only because a liver transplant was performed. In another reported case, a death occurred in a patient with chronic lung disease admitted for a pulmonary infection. From the account, it appears he had been taking only half of his prescribed dose of niacin, so his usual dose was actually doubled when he entered the hospital and received the prescribed amount.

Considering the millions of persons treated around the world in more than 40 years, this experience shows how very infrequent serious liver troubles must be. Nevertheless, it points out two very important precautions: (1) Even though it can be purchased without a prescription, niacin in cholesterol-reducing doses should **not** be self-administered by a patient but must be supervised by a physician. (2) The physician supervising the niacin program should be thoroughly familiar with the use of the drug. In his book outlining use of niacin for patients and physicians, Parsons puts it this way:

Niacin is not a do-it-yourself drug. It requires knowledgeable medical supervision.

Significance of Cholesterol Fractions

Niacin is the only drug which lowers total cholesterol, lowers the "bad" (LDL) cholesterol fraction and raises the "good" (HDL) cholesterol fraction. Recent work seems to show that *plain* niacin might raise HDL cholesterol more effectively than time-release forms.

In 1993 the NCEP "Expert Panel" revised its recommendations to pay more attention to the HDL ("good") cholesterol fraction. The reason is that about one-third of persons who have heart attacks have total cholesterol levels in the "desirable" range (below 200) but a "good" cholesterol fraction which is too low (below 35). The 1993 guidelines also lowered the desirable level of LDL ("bad") cholesterol for persons with known atherosclerotic disease: heart attack, anginal chest pain, coronary bypass or other procedure (such as angioplasty or stent), arterial surgery in the neck or legs. The goal for LDL levels in such patients became *less than 100* instead of less than 130. The reason for this change was that during the previous ten years there had been about ten studies which showed that aggressive reduction of LDL cholesterol results not only in retardation of new cholesterol plaques in arteries but also in reduction in size (regression) of existing deposits. This has been accomplished in a number of ways, including combining niacin with another agent.

If you have any questions about treatment of hypercholesteremia, please let me know. Good luck as we work together to manage your cholesterol problems with niacin!

APPENDIX B

Conversion Table

U.S. System (milligrams per deciliter, mg/dl or mg%) to S.I. System (millimols per liter, mm/L)

U.S. (mg/dl)	S.I. (mm/L)	Comments
400	10.34	Multiply U.S. units by 0.02586 for SI units.
350	9.05	Multiply SI units by 38.7 for U.S. units.
300	7.76	
270	6.98	
240	6.21	Total cholesterol (TC) too high above this level
220	5.69	
200	5.20	TC desirable below this level
160	4.14	If 0-1 risk factors, LDLC satisfactory below this level
130	3.36	If 2 or more risk factors, LDLC satisfactory below this level
100	2.59	If previous event, LDLC desirable below this level
60	1.56	HDLC excellent above this level
45	1.16	HDLC desirable above this level
35	0.91	HDLC dangerous below this level

INDEX

Give the Gift of

Cholesterol Control Without Diet!
The Niacin Solution

to Your Doctor, Friends and Loved Ones

CHECK YOUR LEADING BOOKSTORE OR ORDER HERE

❑ **YES**, I want ____ copies of *Cholesterol Control Without Diet! The Niacin Solution* at $19.95 each, plus $3 shipping per book (Arizona residents please add $1.00 sales tax per book). Canadian orders must be accompanied by a postal money order in U.S. funds. Allow 15 days for delivery.

My check or money order for $_____ is enclosed.
Please charge my ❑ Visa   ❑ MasterCard

Name _____

Organization _____

Address _____

City/State/Zip _____

Phone _____

Credit Card Number _____

Exp. date_____ Signature _____

Please make your check payable and return to:

Lilac Press
P.O. Box 1356
Scottsdale, AZ 85252-1356

Or call your credit card orders to:
(800) 852-4890